DOPPLER ECHOCARDI

THE QUANTITATIVE APPROACH

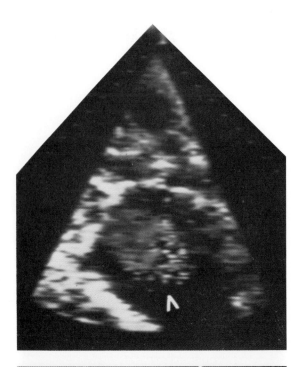

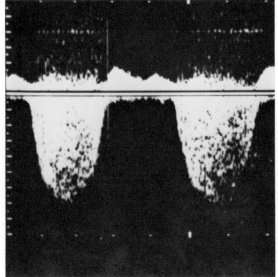

DOPPLER ECHOCARDIOGRAPHY

THE QUANTITATIVE APPROACH

Arthur J. Labovitz, MD, FACC
Associate Professor of Medicine
St. Louis University School of Medicine
Director Echocardiography and
    Noninvasive Hemodynamics
St. Louis, Missouri

George A. Williams, MD, FACC
Associate Professor of Medicine
St. Louis University School of Medicine
Chief, Cardiology Section
VA Medical Center
St. Louis, Missouri

Second Edition

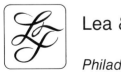 Lea & Febiger

Philadelphia   1988

Lea & Febiger
600 Washington Square
Philadelphia, PA   19106-4198
U.S.A.
(215) 922-1330

Library of Congress Cataloging-in-Publication Data

Labovitz, Arthur
　Doppler echocardiography.

　1. Ultrasonic cardiography. 2. Heart—Diseases—
Diagnosis. 3. Doppler ultrasonography. I. Williams,
George, 1946–　. II. Title. [DNLM: 1. Echocardiography.
2. Heart Diseases—diagnosis. WG 141.5.E2 L125d]
　RC683.5.U5L33　1987　　　616.1′207544　　　87-3287
　ISBN 0-8121-1105-2

PRINTED IN THE UNITED STATE OF AMERICA

Print No.　4　3　2　1

TO OUR WIVES, TERESE AND MARGE

Preface

It has been almost two years since the printing of the first edition of this workbook on Doppler echocardiography. During these two years the clinical application of Doppler ultrasound in the diagnosis of cardiac diseases has seen unprecedented growth. The application of computer technology to rapidly measure frequency shifts of ultrasonic waves backscattered from red blood cells has enabled descriptions of intracardiac blood flow previously accessible only by invasive means. The additional conversion of these frequency shifts to velocity measurements and subsequent gray scale representations from spectral analysis provides a valuable tool for the clinician in the noninvasive evaluation of cardiac pathology. The Doppler examination has become a routine adjunct in the comprehensive evaluation of valvular as well as congenital heart disease. The ability to perform volumetric measurements such as cardiac output with these techniques has stimulated additional and widespread application of Doppler ultrasound in the evaluation of left ventricular function in a variety of clinical situations including exercise. Real-time two-dimensional color flow Doppler has begun to move from the research laboratory into the clinical arena. Reports over the past two years have indicated that Doppler ultrasound may be the procedure of choice for assessment of left ventricular diastolic function. These rapid changes in our understanding and application of the Doppler effect have made this printing of a second edition necessary.

The underlying objective remains to provide a basic primer in the clinical applications of Doppler ultrasound. This edition is not intended to provide either a comprehensive review of the physical principles involved in Doppler technique or an exhaustive review of the literature. It is designed to provide an introduction to the clinical utility of quantitative intracardiac Doppler in the adult. Key references, as well as examples of most clinically encountered disorders, are presented in a simple straightforward manner. We hope this will serve as a basic framework on which many of your own clinical experiences can build.

Finally, we would like to express our gratitude to those who have contributed both directly and indirectly to this book. Our dedicated technicians, Kathleen Habermehl, Jeanne Nelson, Denise Mrosek, Terry Evans, and Jo Kanter, have provided virtually all the illustrations. Susan Buenger deserves special thanks for her expert secretarial assistance. We are also indebted to our colleagues, cardiology fellows, and students.

St. Louis, Missouri

Arthur J. Labovitz, MD
George A. Williams, MD

Contents

1

Doppler Principles

Basic Physics

An understanding of the basic principles of Doppler is necessary before adequate interpretation of Doppler tracings can be expected.

The Doppler effect is present and is used unconsciously in everyday life. When an object (source) producing sound at a particular frequency (pitch) moves toward the listener, the sound appears to be higher pitched (have a higher frequency) than when the source is at rest. When the source moves away from the listener, the sound appears lower pitched. Thus, one can tell if an automobile is moving nearer or away by the rising or falling pitch of the sound its horn makes.

Christian Johann Doppler quantitated this effect for light waves in 1852 to describe the motions of stars with respect to earth. The principle applies to any kind of wave including sound.

To understand Doppler principles, one needs to understand basic terminology:

Frequency: The number of times per second the sound pressure undergoes a cycle of rise and fall, expressed as cycles per second, or Hertz (1 Hz = 1 cycle/sec).

Wavelength: The distance traveled by sound during one cycle.

The speed of sound depends on the characteristics of the material through which it is passing. For soft tissue, the speed is approximately 1540 meters per second (m/sec).

Frequency and wavelength are therefore related. Since sound energy travels only a fixed distance in one second, the more cycles in a second, the shorter the wavelength (Fig. 1). The relationship is:

(1)   Speed of sound (C) = Frequency (F) $\times$ Wavelength (λ)

If the source of sound is moving, the sound waves it produces still travel through the medium at the characteristic speed. Thus, if the source is moving toward the listener, it is "catching up" with the wave it just generated. The wavelength becomes shorter, and the listener hears a higher frequency. If the source is moving away, the wavelength becomes longer, and the listener hears a lower frequency.

1

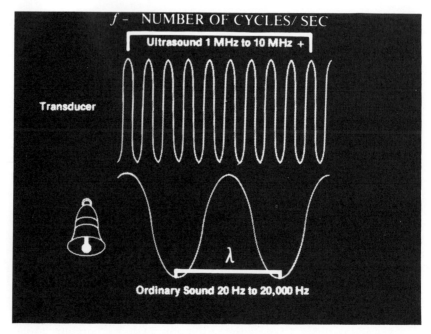

FIGURE 1. Relationship of frequency *(f)* and wavelength (λ). Ordinary sound (bottom), is of low frequency and relatively long wavelength. Ultrasound, "transducer" (top), has a high frequency, since more cycles are present within the same distance, the wavelength is shorter.

The difference between the frequency generated by the source and that observed by the listener is the Doppler shift:

(2) Doppler shift (F_D)

$$= \text{Observed frequency } (F_1) - \text{Original frequency } (F_O)$$

Thus, in ultrasound, if 2,000,000 Hz is sent into the tissue, and 2,006,000 is received (reflected by a moving object), the Doppler shift is +6,000 Hz.

The Doppler shift is proportional to the ratio of the speed of the object to the speed of sound and to the generated frequency:

(3) Doppler shift (F_D)

$$= \frac{\text{Velocity of object (V)}}{\text{Speed of sound (C)}} \times \text{Generated frequency } (F_O)$$

In ultrasound we know the speed of sound, the original (generated) frequency, and the frequency shift, and therefore we can solve for the velocity of red cells (the sound-reflecting objects). To do this, we rearrange the Doppler formula:

(4) $$V = \frac{F_D \times C}{F_O}$$

Doppler's original equation was based on transmitted waveforms only. Since we make use of reflected sound waves, the Doppler shift occurs twice, in the forward and in the reflected wave. To obtain the observed velocity, the formula must be divided by 2:

$$(5) \qquad V = \frac{F_D \times C}{2F_O}$$

Finally, the angle of the transducer must be taken into consideration. If the direction of travel of the transducer beam is not parallel to blood flow, the velocity recorded by the transducer may be an underestimate. This underestimation can be corrected by dividing the formula by the cosine of the angle between the beam and the blood flow:

$$(6) \qquad V = \frac{F_D \times C}{2F_O \times \cos \theta}$$

In practical terms, the best velocity recordings are obtained when the beam is oriented parallel to blood flow ($\cos \theta = 1$). If the beam is 20° off parallel, the error is only 6%, but increasing the angle to 30° increases the error to 13%. Thus, always try to align the Doppler beam to within 20° of blood flow. The approach to Doppler, therefore, is different from echo imaging. In echo the best imaging is obtained when the transducer is perpendicular to structures. In Doppler, the most accurate velocities are recorded with the transducer parallel to blood flow. This will require different viewing windows and techniques, as will be seen.

Doppler Modes

Basically, two Doppler modes are used to examine the heart, both of which have a specific place in the examination of normal and abnormal hearts.

Continuous-Wave Mode

With this technique, two side-by-side transducers (two crystals in one transducer housing) are used. One transducer continuously generates sound waves that travel into the tissue, and the other transducer continuously receives the reflected sound waves. With this method, sound reflections from all depths through which the Doppler beam has passed are simultaneously returning and being analyzed.

Pulsed Wave Mode

In this mode, a single transducer (crystal) emits a short burst of sound energy and awaits the return of reflected sound waves. By analyzing sound received only at specific times (gating), one can localize and analyze reflections from a specific depth. This form of Doppler, called single gate, is the basic technique used to localize and measure normal flow.

Both pulsed- and continuous-wave Doppler have distinct advantages and disadvantages. Continuous-wave Doppler can scan the entire heart very quickly and is used to search for and locate abnormal flow signals. It has a very high velocity limit, but no depth or range resolution (it is unable to localize along the sound beam). Because pulsed-mode Doppler is capable of range resolution, it can be used to define the precise source of abnormal signals. However, it is unable to measure high frequency shifts (high velocities).

The major advantages and disadvantages of each mode are:

	PULSED WAVE MODE	CONTINUOUS-WAVE MODE
Advantages	Range resolution (can interrogate blood flow at a specific depth)	Samples along entire Doppler beam (rapid scanning of heart) Measures high velocities
Disadvantages	Aliasing (cannot measure high velocity)	No range resolution

For pulsed-mode Doppler to accurately measure returning frequencies, the number of pulses generated per second (pulse repetition frequency, or PRF) must be more than twice the frequency of the sound being measured. If the PRF is less than twice the returning frequency, aliasing, an artifactual reversal of velocities occurs. An example of aliasing is seen in Western movies. The camera shutter takes still pictures (samples) 45 times per second. When a stagecoach is moving slowly, its wheels appear to move forward. As it travels faster, however, the spokes on the wheel appear to stop and then rotate backward, as aliasing occurs due to the relationship between their movement and sampling rate of the camera.

Continuous-wave Doppler effectively has an infinite PRF and can therefore measure very high velocities.

Recent modifications of pulsed Doppler include high PRF and multigate techniques. Increasing the PRF to two to four times its normal value raises pulsed-mode velocity limits proportionately, enabling the measurement of higher velocities without aliasing. However, a high PRF increases the number of sampling sites within the heart and introduces the problem of "range ambiguity," the loss of the ability to localize in the pulsed mode. Range ambiguity does not necessarily mean total loss of localization. Although multiple sample sites are present within the heart, they are usually pictured on the two-dimensional image, and typically only one sample volume lies in an area where increased flow velocity is expected. Thus, "localization" can be achieved by placing the appropriate sample volume at the site of the lesion to be interrogated. High-PRF Doppler has been shown to provide useful gradient information in stenotic lesions similar to that obtained from continuous-wave Doppler.

Multigate Doppler is the analysis of several samples along a single line of information. It differs from high-PRF Doppler in that the sample volumes are measured at different times (depth) after transmission of a single burst of ultrasound. Multigate Doppler allows "flow mapping" (see Color Doppler, Chapter 10).

Although phased-array techniques allow "simultaneous" Doppler tracings and two-dimensional imaging, all duplex Doppler systems allow the Doppler cursor line to be superimposed on the two-dimensional image. Phased-array systems "share" imaging and Doppler modes by switching quickly from one to the other. The result is a degradation of both the image and the Doppler signal. For optimal recording of Doppler with phased array, and for real-time Doppler using a mechanical scanner, the image should be frozen. Periodic image "updates" allow localization during the study. The representation of the pulsed-mode sample volume is a box that can be moved up or down on the Doppler cursor. It is important to remember that, although the box represents a sample volume of a fixed length along the line, its width and depth are equal to the size of the ultrasound beam itself. Also, beam width problems that affect imaging can affect a Doppler recording.

"Blind" Doppler nonimaging transducers can be used for intracardiac sampling. Although the lack of an accompanying image is at first disconcerting, these transducers are smaller and in many cases more sensitive than imaging transducers. With practice, nonimaging Doppler can be easier than duplex scanning.

Doppler Tracings

All modern Doppler equipment displays Doppler signals as a spectral tracing: a graph of all the returning signals along a time axis. By convention, velocities of red blood cells traveling toward the transducer are displayed above a zero baseline. Velocities of cells moving away from the transducer are displayed below the baseline. The spectral baseline can be moved up or down to double the velocity limit for unidirectional blood flow (Fig. 2).

A gray scale in the spectral tracing represents the strength of the returning signal by varying shades of gray. Since red blood cells are reflecting the ultrasound, the more cells moving at a certain speed, the stronger the signal for their velocity and the darker its representation on the tracing. The spectral tracing thus gives information about the character of blood flow, by the gray scale, as well as the speed of the majority of cells.

Because all returning velocities are shown on a spectral tracing, information can be obtained about types of blood flow.

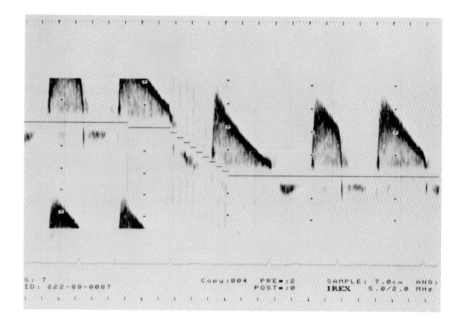

FIGURE 2. Pulsed-mode Doppler tracing of high velocity. The very high portions "wrap around" to the bottom of the panel at left (aliasing). Moving the baseline, at right, allows display of the entire velocity profile as it actually occurs.

Types of Blood Flow

Two basic types of blood flow are distinguished: laminar and nonlaminar.

Laminar

Normal blood flow is called "laminar." All cells are moving in the same direction; but, because they tend to be more densely packed along the walls of vessels, layers (laminae) of blood cells develop. Laminar flow occurs in two patterns: flat and parabolic profiles.

FLAT PROFILE

When blood speeds up (accelerates), all cells tend to move at the same speed. If one could label the cells at a particular cross section and watch their motion, they would appear to be advancing together in a flat front (Figure 3A). Returning Doppler signals would cluster around this velocity with a narrow band on the spectral tracing. A flat flow profile is normally obtained in larger vessels, such as the aorta and the main pulmonary artery near their origins.

PARABOLIC PROFILE

When blood slows down (decelerates), the more densely packed cells at the edges slow down faster than those at the center of the vessel and

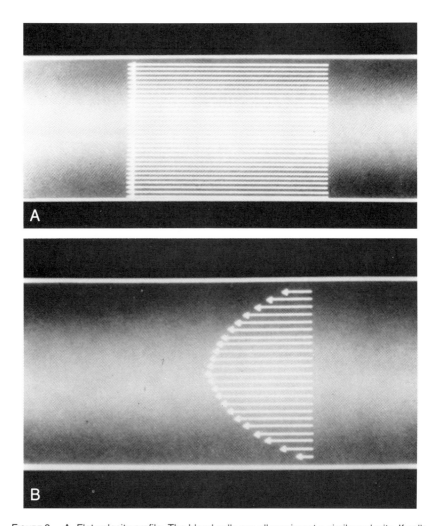

FIGURE 3.   A. Flat velocity profile. The blood cells are all moving at a similar velocity. If cells were marked at the beginning of the arrows, they would all have traveled approximately the same distance in the same time to the arrowheads. B. Parabolic velocity profile. As blood decelerates, the cells at the center of the vessel are retarded less than those at the edges. Thus, if cells are marked at the beginning of the arrows, when they lay in the same plane, central cells would have advanced more than edge cells during a given interval, producing the curved shape at the arrowheads.

the center cells move ahead of their neighbors. Thus, "labeled" cells traveling in a flat profile at one time will present a parabolic profile with a forward bulging center when sampled at a later time (Figure 3B). The spectral tracing will reflect the multiple velocities with a wider band of signals.

Nonlaminar Flow

When the vessel contains an obstruction, blood is forced to flow around it at a faster than normal velocity. Eddies (whirlpools) tend to form distal to the obstruction. The result is nonlaminar flow, the simultaneous movement of blood in multiple directions and at multiple velocities. Nonlaminar flow is also referred to as turbulence.

Summary

Doppler tracings give information about speed, direction, and character of blood flow. The user must keep in mind the problems of angle, beam width, and Doppler mode in adequately performing and interpreting the test.

2

Normal Examination

Technical Considerations

Doppler Display

While simultaneous imaging offers a distinct advantage over the separate Doppler and two-dimensional echo, the user must realize that the best two-dimensional images are obtained with the ultrasound beam perpendicular to structures, while the best Doppler signal is obtained with the beam parallel to flow. Therefore, the best Doppler signal may accompany a less than optimal two-dimensional image. The two basic pieces of information obtained by Doppler are direction and velocity. By convention, most commercially available equipment will display flow toward the transducer above the baseline and flow away from the transducer below the baseline. The spectral display is a gray scale graph of the distribution of velocities in a population of red blood cells.

Doppler Mode

The utility of Doppler systems with both pulsed and continuous-wave capabilities will be emphasized in the evaluation of cardiac pathology. In the "normal" individual, however, velocities in the heart and great vessels should not exceed the velocity limits of the pulsed mode when the baseline shift is used.

Angle of Incidence

To record reproducible quantitative Doppler information, the user should concentrate efforts on making the ultrasound beam as parallel to flow as possible. The major components of the Doppler equation:

$$V = \frac{(F_1 - F_O)(C)}{(2F_O)\,(\cos\theta)}$$

where: V = flow velocity
F_1 = received frequency
F_O = emitted frequency
C = velocity of sound in blood

are automatically calculated by most commercially available equipment. The variable controlled by the user is cos θ, which approximates 1.0 at angles of less than 20°.

Standard Doppler Windows

With few exceptions, the normal adult patient can receive a complete Doppler examination using three standard windows: the cardiac apex, the left parasternal region (short axis view), and the suprasternal notch. Additional information may be obtained in selected cases from the right parasternal and subcostal windows (Figure 4).

Apical Window

MITRAL VALVE

When interrogating the mitral valve from the apical window, place the Doppler transducer at the point of maximal impulse at the cardiac apex. When the sample volume is positioned at the level of the mitral valve, intracardiac blood flow is toward the transducer in diastole (Figure 5). This is demonstrated by a positive displacement of the spectrum in diastole. Some "contamination" by left ventricular outflow tract velocities may be recorded during systole while examining transmitral flow (Figure 6).

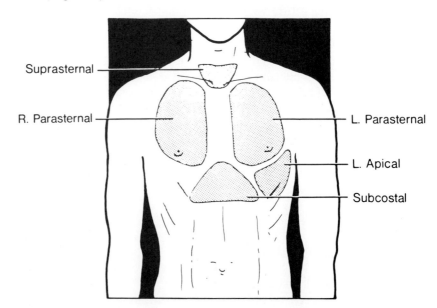

FIGURE 4.   Location of commonly used Doppler examination windows.

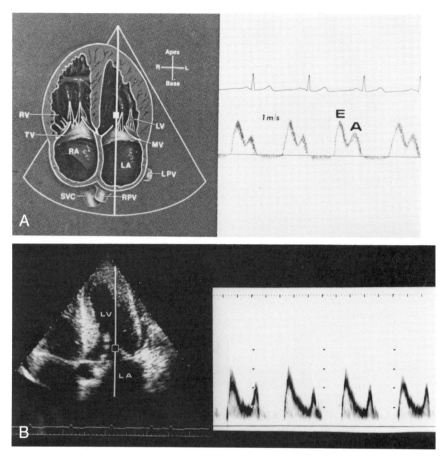

FIGURE 5. Schematic (A) and actual tracing (B) of normal mitral flow. E represents early diastolic filling; A represents atrial systole. The E:A velocity ratio is normally greater than 1.0. Normal range of velocities is 0.4–l.4 m/sec.

TRICUSPID VALVE

When interrogating tricuspid valve flow from the apical window, place the Doppler transducer at the point just medial to the point of maximal impulse at the cardiac apex.

When the sample volume is positioned at the level of the tricuspid valve, intracardiac blood flow is toward the transducer in diastole (Figure 7). This is demonstrated by a positive displacement of the spectrum in diastole. These velocities are increased on inspiration.

LEFT VENTRICULAR OUTFLOW TRACT AND AORTIC VALVE

When interrogating left ventricular outflow tract (LVOT) flow from the apical window, place the Doppler transducer at the point of maximal impulse at the cardiac apex. Pulsed-mode Doppler can be used to sample the flows in the areas of interest.

When the sample volume is positioned in the LVOT, below the aortic valve, intracardiac blood flow is away from the transducer in systole.

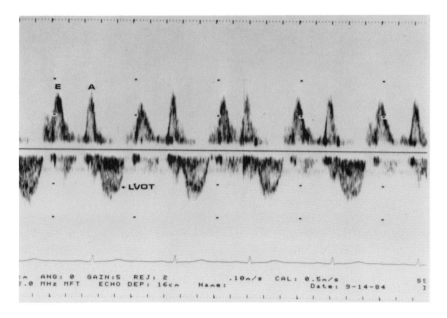

FIGURE 6. Both left ventricular inflow (E and A) as well as left ventricular outflow tract (LVOT) are commonly seen when examining transmitral flow.

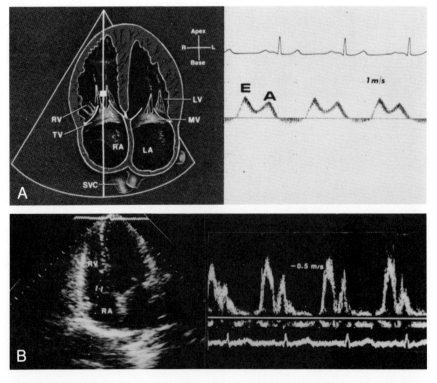

FIGURE 7. Schematic (A) and actual tracing (B) of normal tricuspid flow. E represents early diastolic filling; A represents atrial systole. Normal range of velocities is 0.3–1.0 m/sec.

This is demonstrated by a negative displacement of the spectrum in systole (Figure 8). Systolic velocities will be noted to progressively increase from the papillary muscle level to the aortic valve.

Left Parasternal Window: Short Axis View

PULMONIC VALVE

When interrogating the pulmonic valve from the left parasternal window, place the transducer in the third or fourth intercostal space on the left side of the sternum. Obtain the short axis view of the aorta and aim the transducer slightly superiorly and laterally. Pulsed-mode Doppler can be used to sample blood flow at the area of interest.

When the sample volume is positioned at the level of the pulmonic valve, intracardiac blood flow is away from the transducer in systole (Figure 9). This is demonstrated by a negative displacement of the spectrum in systole.

TRICUSPID VALVE

When interrogating the tricuspid valve from the left parasternal window in the short axis, place the transducer at the third or fourth intercostal space on the left side of the sternum. Obtain a short axis view of the aorta and aim the transducer medially for the tricuspid valve. It should be noted that a long axis view of the tricuspid valve can also be obtained from this window. After obtaining a standard long axis view of the aortic and mitral valves, aim the transducer medially to obtain the long axis of the right ventricular inflow tract. Either the apical or parasternal view is acceptable for Doppler of the tricuspid valve. Pulsed-mode Doppler can be used to sample areas of interest.

When the sample volume is positioned at the level of the tricuspid

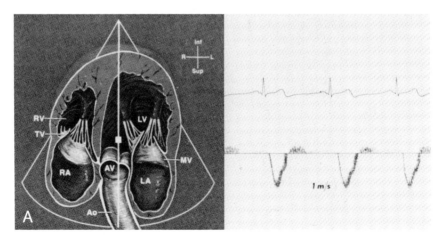

FIGURE 8. Schematic (A) and representative tracing (B) of normal left ventricular outflow tract velocities. The velocities increase progressively from the body of the left ventricle to the aortic valve level. Normal velocity range is 0.5–1.8 m/sec.

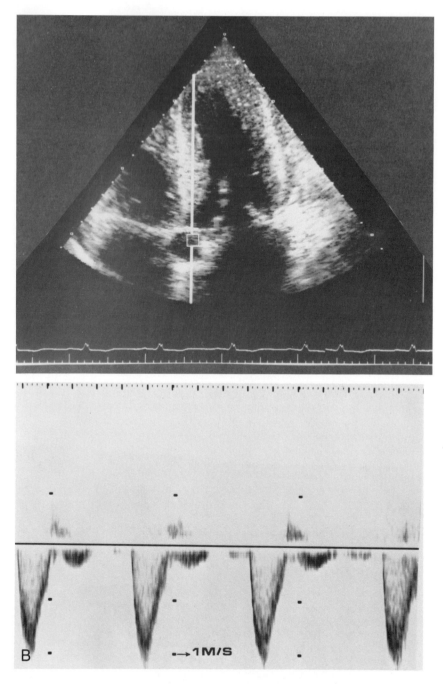

FIGURE 8 (continued).

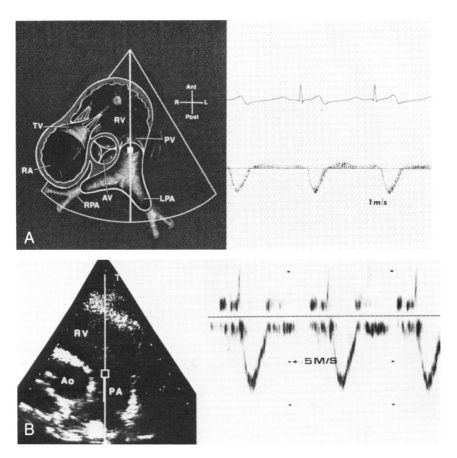

FIGURE 9. Schematic (A) and representative tracing (B) of normal pulmonary artery flow. Normal velocity range is 0.5–1.5 m/sec.

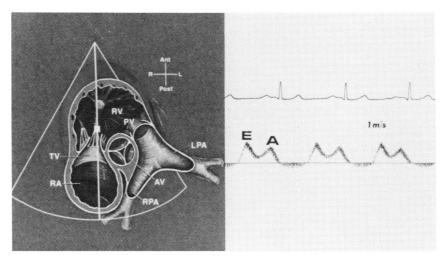

FIGURE 10. Tricuspid valve flow from the short axis view. Normal velocity range is 0.3– 1.0 m/sec. E represents early diastolic filling; A represents atrial systole.

valve, intracardiac blood flow is toward the transducer in diastole (Figure 10). This is demonstrated by a positive displacement of the spectrum in diastole. Spectral recording is similar to that obtained from the cardiac apex.

Suprasternal Notch Window

ASCENDING AORTA

When interrogating the ascending aorta from the suprasternal notch, aim the transducer toward the heart in the short axis plane. Pulsed mode can be used to sample the area of interest. It should be noted that, because of the large transducer size, it is sometimes impossible to use an imaging and Doppler probe in the suprasternal notch. The smaller independent Doppler transducer is quicker to use and more comfortable for the patient.

When the sample volume is positioned in the ascending aorta, blood flow is toward the transducer in systole (Figure 11). This is demonstrated by a positive displacement of the spectrum in systole.

DESCENDING AORTA

When interrogating the descending aorta from the suprasternal notch, aim the transducer toward the heart in the short axis plane. Pulsed mode can be used to sample the area of interest. It should be noted that, because of the large transducer size, it is sometimes impossible to use an imaging and Doppler transducer in the suprasternal notch. The smaller independent Doppler transducer is quicker to use and more comfortable for the patient.

When the sample volume is positioned in the descending aorta, blood flow is away from the transducer in systole (Figure 12). This is demonstrated by a negative displacement in the spectrum in systole.

Nonstandard Doppler Windows

Right Parasternal Window

ASCENDING AORTA

When interrogating the ascending aorta from the right parasternal window, place the transducer in the second, third, or fourth intercostal space on the right side of the sternum. The best signals are obtained with the patient lying right side down and with an independent Doppler transducer. The continuous-mode can be used to quickly locate the best angle of incidence and best assessment of flow velocities.

When the sample volume is positioned in the ascending aorta, blood flow is toward the transducer in systole. This is demonstrated by a positive displacement of the spectrum. This view is extremely useful

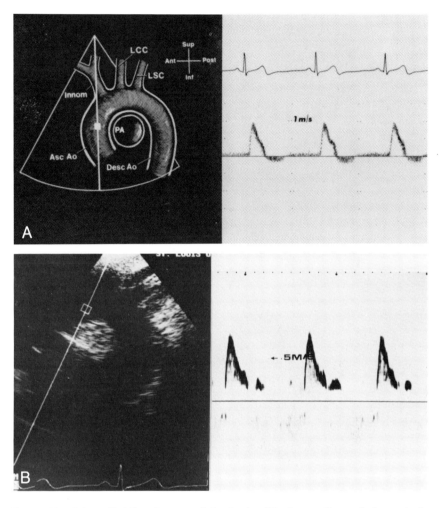

FIGURE 11. Schematic (A) and representative tracing (B) of ascending aortic flow velocity from the suprasternal notch. Normal range is 0.5–1.5 m/sec.

in evaluating aortic valve flow in patients with aortic stenosis (see Aortic Valve Pathology, Chapter 4).

Subcostal Window

When interrogating the heart from the subcostal window, place the transducer just below the costal area, aimed superiorly and laterally toward the heart.

This window is often used with patients who have chronic lung disease or for whom examination from conventional windows is technically difficult. Both inflow and outflow valves can be interrogated from this window with the ultrasound beam not quite parallel to the flow. This window can also be used to evaluate atrial septal defects. The continuous wave can be used to locate the best angle of incidence

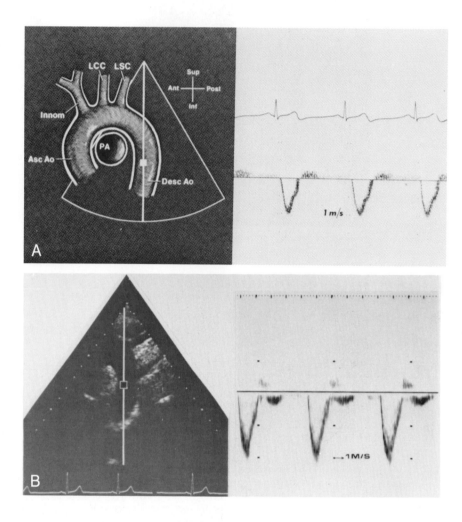

FIGURE 12.   Schematic (A) and representative tracing (B) of descending aortic flow velocity from the suprasternal notch. Normal range is 0.5–1.5 m/sec.

and best flow velocity, and the pulsed mode used to sample a specific area of interest.

Left Parasternal Window: Long Axis View

Because of difficulty in examining aortic and mitral flow in a parallel fashion from this view, quantitative measurements are not recommended. However, qualitative information about mitral or aortic insufficiency is still possible (Figures 13, 14).

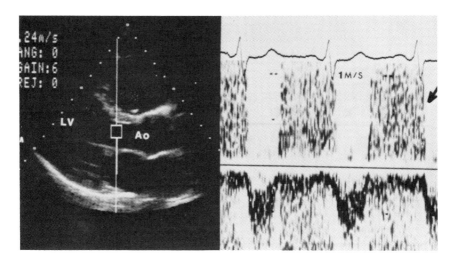

FIGURE 13. Parasternal long axis view with the sample volume positioned in the left ventricular outflow tract. Aortic insufficiency (arrow) is clearly seen.

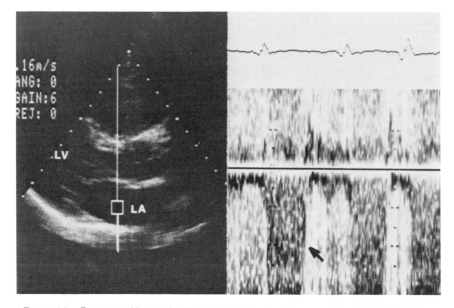

FIGURE 14. Parasternal long axis view with the sample volume positioned in the left atrium. Holosystolic jet of mitral regurgitation (arrow) is evident.

References

Grenadier, E., Lima, C.O., Allen, H.D., Sahn, D.J., Barron, J.V., Valdes-Cruz, L.M., and Goldberg, S.J.: Normal intracardiac and great vessel Doppler flow velocities in infants and children. JACC, *4*:343–350, 1984.

Loeber, C.P., Goldberg, S.J., and Allen, H.D.: Doppler echocardiographic comparison of flows distal to the four cardiac valves. JACC, *4*:268–272, 1984.

3

Calculations

Two major Doppler calculations are made to interpret abnormal signals: the modified Bernoulli equation and pressure halftime. The derivation of these formulas will be explained here and clinical applications described in the following chapters.

Bernoulli Equation

The Bernoulli equation for fluid flow past an obstruction is a relationship between the pressures before and after the obstruction (P_1, P_2), the properties of the fluid, such as the density (ρ), the fluid velocities before and after the obstruction (V_1, V_2), and quantities that depend on the type of fluid and type of obstruction. These quantities involve the flow acceleration, expressed mathematically in terms from differential calculus as the summation (integral) of small increments (dV is an increment of velocity, dt of time, and ds of distance), and the viscous friction, $R(V)$, acting to retard the flow. The complete equation is:

(1)
$$P_1 - P_2 = \tfrac{1}{2}\rho\,(V_2^2 - V_1^2) + \rho \int_1^2 \frac{dV}{dt}\,ds + R(V)$$

$$\underset{\text{change)}}{\text{(Pressure}} = \underset{\text{acceleration)}}{\text{(Convective}} + \underset{\text{acceleration)}}{\text{(Flow}} + \underset{\text{forces)}}{\text{(Friction}}$$

This unwieldy formula is simplified for clinical use by making two assumptions: 1) If we use maximal velocity, flow acceleration is 0 (zero), and 2) In stenotic valves the diameter of the orifice is wide in relation to the length, which, by Pouiselle's Law, makes the friction forces very small until the diameter of the valve orifice is less than 2 mm, a condition not seen in life. Thus, in general, friction forces and flow acceleration can be ignored, leaving only convective forces. With the density of blood expressed in appropriate units, the equation then becomes:

(2)
$$P_1 - P_2 \text{ (mmHg)} = 4(V_2^2 - V_1^2)$$

When V_1 is less than 1 m/sec, it can be ignored, leaving:

(3)
$$P_1 - P_2 = 4V_{max}^2 \text{ (Figure 15)}$$

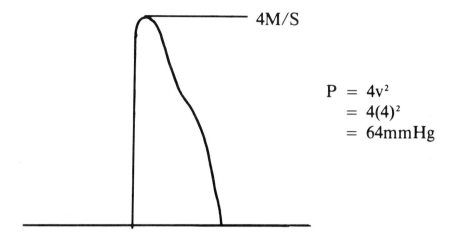

$$P = 4v^2$$
$$= 4(4)^2$$
$$= 64mmHg$$

FIGURE 15. Application of Bernoulli's principle to a high velocity jet. The peak velocity of 4 m/sec is squared and then multiplied by 4 to obtain the pressure gradient in mm Hg.

Mean Gradient

The mean pressure gradient is calculated by measuring the velocity at equally spaced points, squaring each velocity, averaging the squared velocity values, and multiplying the average by 4 (Figure 16).

Pressure Halftime

When blood flows passively through a stenotic valve, the size of the valve opening (orifice) can be estimated from the amount of time it takes the initial peak pressure gradient to fall to one-half (pressure halftime, $P_{1/2}$) its original value. This can be done from the Doppler tracing as follows:

1. Measure the initial peak velocity from the tracing and draw a vertical line from the peak to the horizontal axis (Figure 17). Never include the outline of the "A" wave velocity.

2. The velocity at the time the pressure gradient has fallen to half its initial value can be shown to be approximately $V_{max}/1.4$. The quantity 1.4 is approximately the square root of 2. Since pressure difference is related to V^2, the derivation of the V corresponding to $P_{1/2}$ involves taking square roots, including the square root of 2. Therefore, divide the peak velocity by 1.4 (Figure 18) and mark this point on the vertical line drawn in step 1. Draw a horizontal line through the point (Figure 19).

3. To estimate $P_{1/2}$, first draw a sloping line along the top of the tracing (maximum velocities) until it intersects the horizontal line drawn in step 2, then draw a vertical line down from the intersection. Now measure the distance between the two vertical lines and determine the time interval it represents from the timing marks at the edge of the

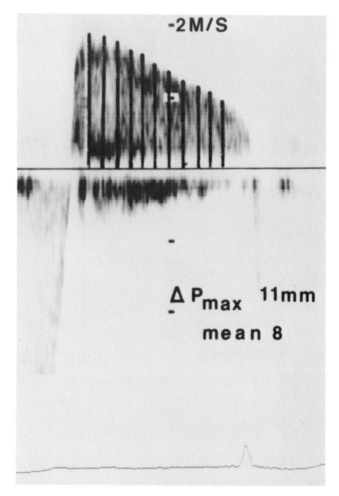

FIGURE 16. Calculation of mean pressure gradient. Velocities are measured at multiple points, values are squared, and the mean square velocity is used in the modified Bernoulli equation.

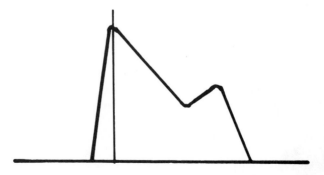

FIGURE 17. Maximum velocity is measured from tracing and vertical line is drawn through peak.

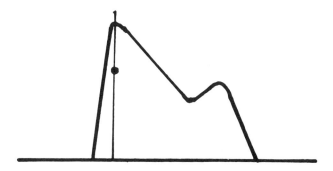

FIGURE 18. Point is marked on vertical at level equal to $V_{max}/1.4$.

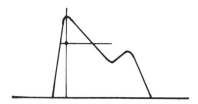

FIGURE 19. Horizontal line is drawn through point at $V_{max}/1.4$.

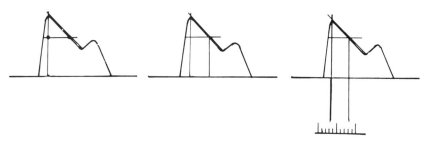

FIGURE 20. Determination of pressure halftime. Horizontal distance on tracing between V_{max} and $V_{max}/1.4$ points is measured and gauged against time scale.

tracing (Figure 20). This interval is the pressure halftime in milliseconds.

4. An estimate of the valve orifice area is based on the fact that $P_{1/2}$ remains relatively constant for a given orifice area over a wide range of flows. For an orifice area of 1 cm², $P_{1/2}$ is 220 milliseconds. The effective orifice area is therefore:

$$\text{Orifice area} = 220/P_{1/2} \text{ cm}^2$$

References

Hatle, L.: Non-invasive assessment and differentiation of left ventricular outflow obstruction with Doppler ultrasound. Circulation 4:380–388, 1981.

Hatle, L., Angelsen, B., and Tromsdal, A.: Non-invasive assessment of atrio-ventricular pressure halftime by Doppler ultrasound. Circulation 60:1096–1104, 1969.

Hatle, L., Angelsen, B., and Tromsdal, A.: Non-invasive assessment of aortic stenosis by Doppler ultrasound. Br. Heart J., 43:284–292, 1980.

Holen, J., Aaslid, R., Landmark, K., Simonsen, S., and Ostrem, T.: Determination of effective orifice area in mitral stenosis from non-invasive ultrasound Doppler data and mitral flow rate. Acta Med. Scand., 201:83–88, 1977.

Holen, J., Aaslid, R., Landmark, L., and Simonsen, S.: Determination of pressure gradient in mitral stenosis with a noninvasive ultrasound Doppler technique. Acta Med. Scand., 199:455–460, 1976.

Libanoff, A.J., and Rodbard, S.: Atrioventricular pressure halftime measure of mitral valve orifice area. Circulation 38:144–150, 1968.

4

Aortic Valve Pathology

Aortic Stenosis

At the present time, the Doppler evaluation of a stenotic aortic valve is this technology's most popular clinical application. While two-dimensional echocardiography has been disappointing in the assessment of the severity of aortic stenosis, continuous-wave and high-PRF Doppler have been shown in recent reports to yield accurate quantitation of transvalvular gradients. Such quantitation is possible because the velocity of blood flow increases in proportion to the degree of stenosis. The transvalvular gradient can be calculated using the modified Bernoulli equation:

$$Gradient = 4V_{max}^2$$

where V_{max} is the maximal transvalvular aortic velocity (Figure 21). There are, however, some key points the user must keep in mind in the Doppler evaluation of a stenotic aortic valve.

Angle of Incidence

The direction of flow through a calcified stenotic aortic valve is difficult, if not impossible, to guess from the two-dimensional image alone (Figure 22). Because of this, all potentially stenotic aortic valves should be examined from at least three windows to obtain parallelism between the ultrasound beam and the flow: cardiac apex, right parasternal border, and suprasternal notch (Figure 23). The highest velocity obtained from all windows interrogated should be used for V_{max} in the modified Bernoulli equation. Examination from the subcostal window may also be of value.

Peak Instantaneous Gradients

Traditionally, at cardiac catheterization, "peak" pressure gradients are determined by subtracting the peak aortic pressure from the peak

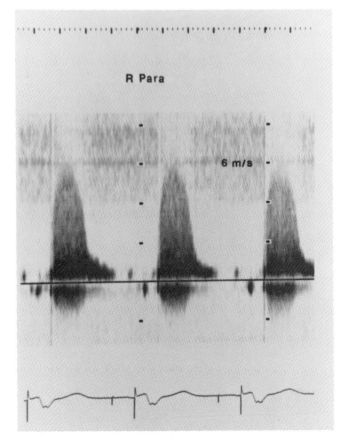

FIGURE 21. Characteristic continuous-wave Doppler tracing from the right parasternal window in a patient with severe aortic stenosis. Calculation by the modified Bernoulli equation would indicate a peak gradient of approximately 144 mm Hg.

STENOTIC JET

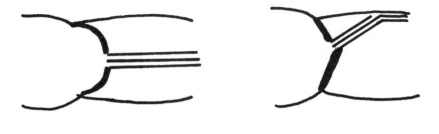

IDEAL   **DEFORMED VALVE**

FIGURE 22. Ideally, to acquire Doppler velocity information with the beam parallel to the flow, the stenotic jet should be oriented parallel to the vessel walls. Unfortunately, the jet through a stenotic aortic valve frequently has an eccentric orientation.

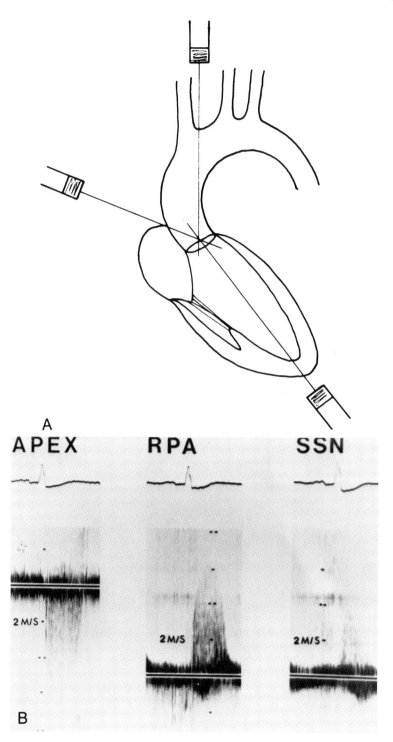

A

APEX   **RPA**   **SSN**

2 M/S ·

2 M/S   2 M/S -

B

FIGURE 23.   (A) All patients suspected of having aortic stenosis should be examined from the cardiac apex, right parasternal, and suprasternal notch windows. (B) In this individual with a gradient of over 100 mm Hg, documented at cardiac catheterization, the suprasternal notch (SSN) recording greatly underestimates the peak velocity shown most clearly from the right parasternal window (RPA).

left ventricular pressure ("peak-to-peak gradients"). Doppler, on the other hand, measures the "peak-instantaneous" gradient (Figure 24).

In cases of moderate to severe aortic stenosis, the difference between the peak-instantaneous and peak-to-peak gradients is minimal, as the peak left ventricular pressure occurs later in systole. However, in cases of mild aortic stenosis, or conditions such as aortic insufficiency in which the velocity in the left ventricular outflow tract (LVOT) may be elevated, significant differences may exist between the peak-instantaneous and peak-to-peak gradients, calculated by the modified Bernoulli equation. These differences can be minimized by using the more complete Bernoulli equation:

$$\text{Gradient} = 4(V^2_{max} - V^2_{LVOT})$$

where V_{max} is the maximal transvalvular aortic velocity, usually measured by continuous-wave Doppler, and V_{LVOT} is the velocity in the left ventricular outflow tract, as measured by pulsed Doppler.

For example, if V_{max} is 3.5 m/sec, and V_{LVOT} is 1.7 m/sec, the "true" transvalvular pressure gradient would be:

$$
\begin{aligned}
\text{Gradient} &= 4[(3.5)^2 - (1.7)^2)] \\
&= 4(12 - 3) \\
&= 4 \times 9 \\
&= 36 \text{ mm Hg}
\end{aligned}
$$

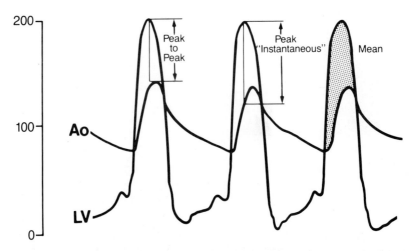

FIGURE 24. The pressure gradient between the aorta (Ao) and left ventricle (LV) has traditionally been reported at cardiac catheterization as the difference between the peak left ventricle and peak aortic pressures (peak to peak) while Doppler measures the peak instantaneous difference. The mean pressure gradient represents the average pressure gradient throughout systole.

Mean transvalvular pressure gradients can also be calculated from the Doppler tracing, by averaging the measured instantaneous gradient every 40 milliseconds, and have been shown to correlate well with invasively measured mean gradients.

Aortic Valve Area

While most cardiologists will agree that a peak-to-peak transvalvular gradient greater than 50 mm Hg represents significant aortic stenosis, the finding of a gradient less than 50 mm Hg does not rule out such a condition. In fact, in the presence of severe left ventricular dysfunction, a gradient of 30 mm Hg may represent critical aortic stenosis. It is, therefore, suggested that a report of the measured aortic valve gradient be coupled with some estimation of left ventricular function from the two-dimensional study.

Several Doppler formulas incorporating an index of left ventricular function have been reported by which aortic valve area may be estimated. In general, these equations have been derived from either the Gorlin or the continuity equation. A simple formula for calculating aortic valve area (AVA), derived from the continuity equation, incorporates the cross-sectional area (CSA) of the aortic valve anulus as well as V_{max} and V_{LVOT}:

$$AVA = \frac{V_{LVOT}}{V_{max}} \times CSA$$

Time to Peak Velocity

The measurement of the time to peak velocity provides additional qualitative information. In normal individuals, Doppler tracings show that the peak aortic velocity usually occurs in the first third of the systolic ejection period. In patients with aortic stenosis, peak velocity usually occurs later and is frequently delayed until the halfway point in the systolic ejection period (Figure 25).

Hypertrophic Cardiomyopathy

Patients with outflow tract obstruction secondary to hypertrophic cardiomyopathy (HCM) will also have high velocity jets seen by continuous-wave Doppler. However, when pulsed Doppler from the cardiac apex is used in evaluating these patients, the increased velocity will be localized to an intraventricular site. Figure 26 shows a parasternal M-mode echocardiogram (A) and a continuous-wave Doppler study from the cardiac apex (B) for a patient with a documented intraventricular gradient of 65 mm Hg. Note the thick septum and the anterior systolic motion of the mitral valve on the M-mode. The Doppler spectral

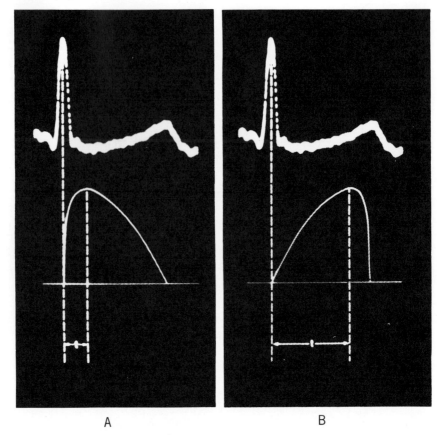

A   B

FIGURE 25.   In normal individuals (A) the peak aortic velocity occurs during the first third of the systolic ejection period, while in patients with aortic stenosis (B) peak velocity may be delayed until much later into the systolic ejection period.

display shows the characteristic concave appearance of the high velocity jet associated with obstructive HCM. Pulsed Doppler localized the obstruction to a region 2 cm proximal to the aortic valve. It has been shown that the timing of the peak anterior motion of the mitral valve correlates with the timing of peak velocity seen by Doppler. Examination of these patients from the ascending aorta will reveal that most of the aortic flow occurs prior to the occurrence of the peak velocity. Care should be taken to distinguish between the high velocity LVOT jet and the high velocity jet of mitral regurgitation commonly seen in these patients (Figure 27).

Aortic Insufficiency

M-mode and two-dimensional echocardiography can be helpful in the etiology but not the qualitative and quantitative analysis of aortic insufficiency. Doppler, however, appears to be exquisitely sensitive in the evaluation of aortic insufficiency. The characteristic Doppler tracing of aortic insufficiency includes two important features: (1) a diastolic

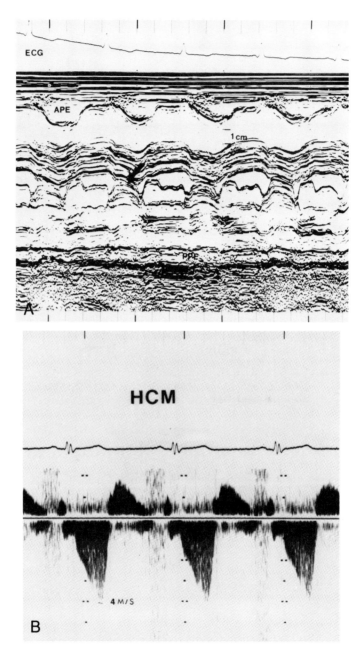

FIGURE 26. (A) M-mode echocardiographic tracing from patient with hypertrophic cardio-myopathy. Note the marked septal hypertrophy and systolic anterior motion of the mitral valve. (B) Typical continuous-wave Doppler tracing from the cardiac apex in patients with hypertrophic cardiomyopathy (HMC). The high velocity intracavitary jet causes a character-istic concave appearance and late systolic peak.

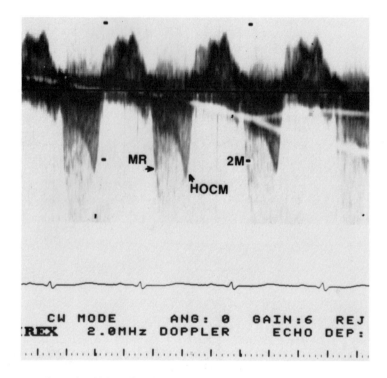

FIGURE 27. Care should be taken in distinguishing between the high velocity jets of left ventricular outflow (HOCM) and mitral regurgitation (MR) commonly seen in these patients.

flow reversal greater than 2 m/sec from aorta to left ventricle and (2) increased systolic aortic velocities in the presence of normal left ventricular systolic function.

Several Doppler methods have been reported to be useful in the quantitation of aortic insufficiency, including flow mapping (pulsed), regurgitant fractions, continuous wave, and real time (color) Doppler.

Pulsed-Doppler Flow Mapping

The most extensively used method in the quantitation of aortic insufficiency by Doppler is flow mapping. With this method, the diastolic jet of aortic insufficiency is "mapped" back into the left ventricle, proximal to the aortic valve, by pulsed Doppler from the apical or parasternal window (Figure 28).

If an insufficient jet extends less than 2 cm from the aortic valve plane into the left ventricle, the insufficiency is considered mild; if the jet is mapped between 2 cm and the papillary muscle level, the insufficiency is considered moderate; and if the jet is beyond the papillary muscle level, the insufficiency is considered severe. Quantitation of the degree of insufficiency by this technique compares well with angiography (Figure 29).

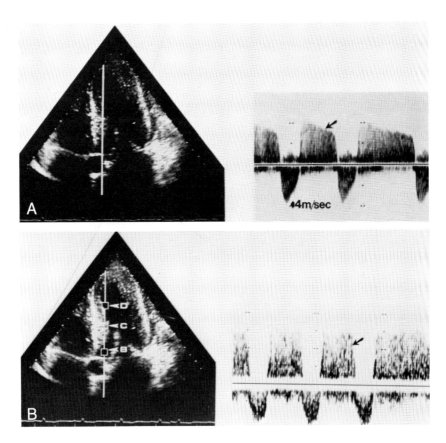

FIGURE 28. Demonstration of pulsed-Doppler mapping technique. Arrows denote regurgitant jet in the continuous mode (A) and at various levels in pulsed Doppler (B–D). In this patient the regurgitant jet extends back to the papillary muscle level, suggesting a moderate degree of insufficiency.

Regurgitant Fractions

A promising method of quantitating the severity of aortic insufficiency is calculation of the regurgitant fraction from the difference between forward stroke volume measured at the aortic valve (AoSV) and forward stroke volume measured at a remote site such as the pulmonic valve (PSV). The regurgitant fraction (RF) can be calculated by the equation:

$$RF = \frac{AoSV - PSV}{AoSV}$$

Regurgitant fractions greater than 25% should be considered significant.

Continuous-Wave Doppler

Recent studies have suggested that the degree of aortic insufficiency may be quantitated from the slope of the aortic insufficient velocities

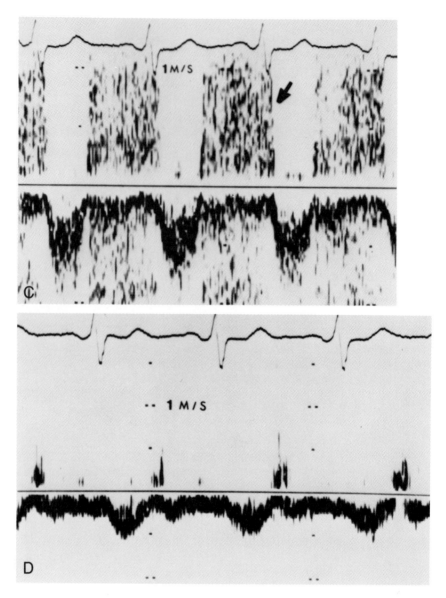

F<small>IGURE</small> 28 (continued).

in continuous-wave Doppler (Figure 30). The principle is that the more severe the insufficiency, the more rapidly will aortic and ventricular pressures equilibrate, and hence the steeper the slope. Slopes greater than 2 m/sec² are usually associated with moderate to severe insufficiency.

Real-Time (Color) Doppler

The use of real-time two-dimensional (color) Doppler has been reported to be useful in assessing the degree of insufficiency from the extent of the insufficient jet into the left ventricle (Figure 31).

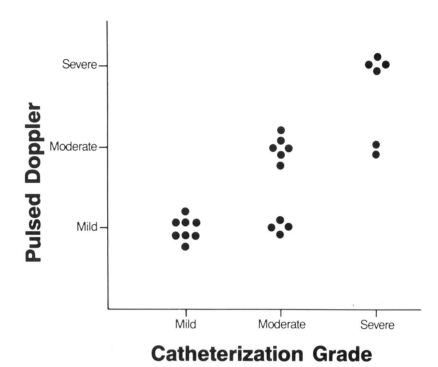

FIGURE 29. Comparison between pulsed-Doppler mapping and angiographic estimation of the degree of aortic insufficiency.

Aortic Valve Pathology Case Studies

Case #1

HISTORY AND PHYSICAL EXAMINATION

A 62-year-old man was admitted to the hospital for evaluation of a syncopal episode. He denied symptoms of chest pain or dyspnea on exertion. On physical examination, a harsh grade IV/VI systolic ejection murmur was heard at the left sternal border with radiation to both carotids. Carotid upstroke was delayed.

ECHOCARDIOGRAPHY AND DOPPLER FINDINGS

The aortic root and valve were heavily calcified and valve opening diminished. The left ventricle appeared to be hypertrophied with relatively normal systolic function. The continuous-wave Doppler tracing obtained from the cardiac apex is shown in Figure 32A, and the pulsed-Doppler tracing from the LVOT is shown in Figure 32B. The diameter of the aortic valve anulus was 2.4 cm, so the cross-sectional area was $\pi (2.4/2)^2 = 4.5$ cm^2, where π is approximately 3.14.

What is the diagnosis? _____
What is the peak gradient? _____
What is the valve area? _____

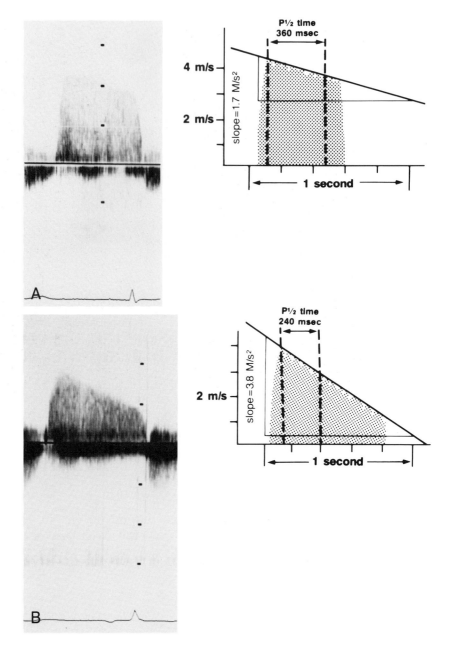

FIGURE 30. Continuous-wave Doppler tracings from (A) a patient with mild aortic insufficiency and (B) a patient with severe aortic insufficiency. Note that the slope is greater and the pressure halftime ($P_{1/2}$) shorter in the patient with severe insufficiency.

ANSWER

This case illustrates typical Doppler findings in severe aortic stenosis. Because the outflow tract velocities were less than 1 m/sec (0.7 m/sec), the simplified Bernoulli equation can be used to calculate the peak aortic transvalvular gradient from the maximum velocity of 5 m/sec:

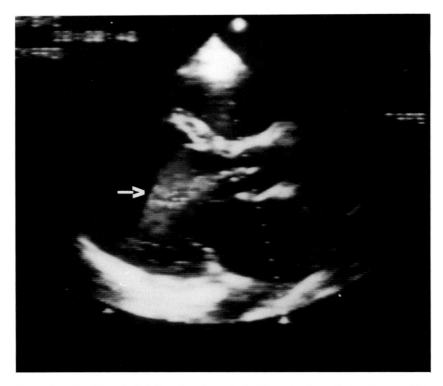

FIGURE 31. Real-time (color) Doppler of a patient with moderate aortic insufficiency. Note the blue jet of aortic insufficiency (arrow) extending well into the left ventricle during diastole.

$$\text{Gradient} = 4\ V_{\text{max}}^2 = 4 \times 25 = 100\ \text{mm Hg}$$

The aortic valve area is calculated from the equation:

$$\text{AVA} = \frac{V_{\text{LVOT}}}{V_{\text{max}}} \times \text{CSA} = \frac{0.7}{5} \times 4.5 = 0.6\ \text{cm}$$

The gradient was subsequently confirmed at cardiac catheterization, and the aortic valve was successfully replaced.

Case #2

HISTORY AND PHYSICAL EXAMINATION

The patient was a 38-year-old tall, thin, white male with long extremities, referred for evaluation of fever and progressive dyspnea on exertion. An older brother had required aortic valve replacement some years earlier for unknown reasons. Carotid upstroke was brisk with a rapid drop-off. Examination of the heart revealed a dynamic cardiac impulse. A diastolic blowing murmur was clearly heard at the second right intercostal space. A systolic ejection murmur was heard at the lower left sternal border.

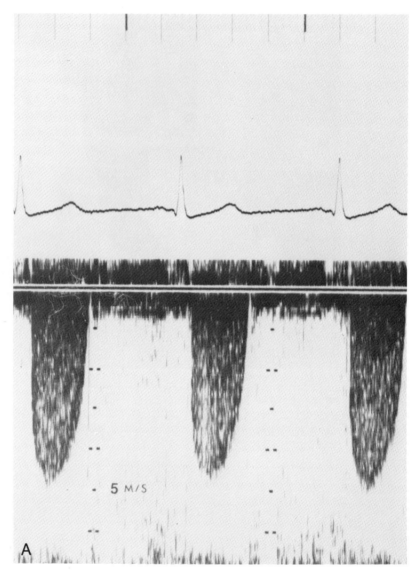

FIGURE 32.

ECHOCARDIOGRAPHY AND DOPPLER FINDINGS

M-mode and 2-dimensional echocardiography revealed an enlarged hyperdynamic left ventricle. The aortic valve leaflets were thin, with a prolapsing mass seen on the noncoronary cusp (arrow, Figure 33A). Mild mitral valve prolapse was also seen. The continuous-wave Doppler tracing made from the cardiac apex is shown in Figure 33B. Pulsed-Doppler recordings are shown from the LVOT (Figure 33C) and papillary muscle level (Figure 33D).

What is the diagnosis? _____

Is there significant aortic insufficiency? _____

What is the aortic transvalvular gradient? _____

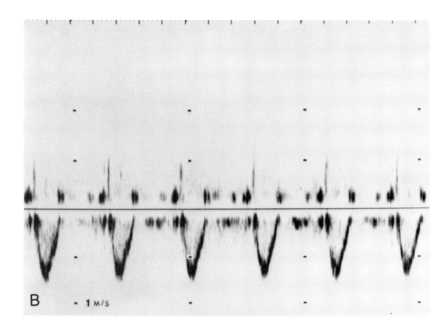

Figure 32 (continued).

ANSWER

A prominent high velocity diastolic jet of aortic insufficiency is seen from the cardiac apex in continuous-wave Doppler. The slope of velocity decay is quite steep, suggesting a significant degree of insufficiency. This jet was shown by pulsed Doppler to extend to the level of the papillary muscles, indicating a moderate degree of regurgitation. The velocity in the LVOT was approximately 1.5 m/sec, indicating that, despite a 2.0-m/sec systolic velocity seen in the continuous wave mode, minimal if any aortic valve gradient was present. Applying the more extensive Bernoulli equation:

$$\text{Gradient} = 4(V_2^2 - V_1^2)$$
$$= 4[(2.0)^2 - (1.5)^2]$$
$$= 7 \text{ mm Hg}$$

Blood cultures obtained on admission grew Staphylococcus aureus, confirming the diagnosis of bacterial endocarditis.

Case #3

HISTORY AND PHYSICAL EXAMINATION

A 68-year-old man admitted to the hospital for a urologic procedure was noted to have a heart murmur on physical examination. He denied symptoms referable to the cardiovascular system. Consultation was obtained with the cardiology service. On physical examination, a Grade III/VI systolic ejection murmur was heard at the aortic area. A soft

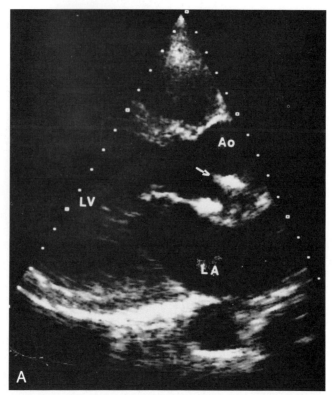

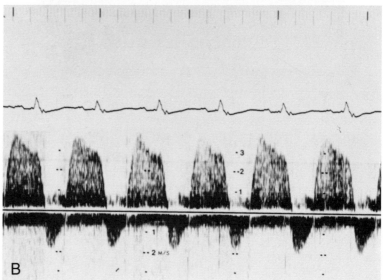

FIGURE 33.

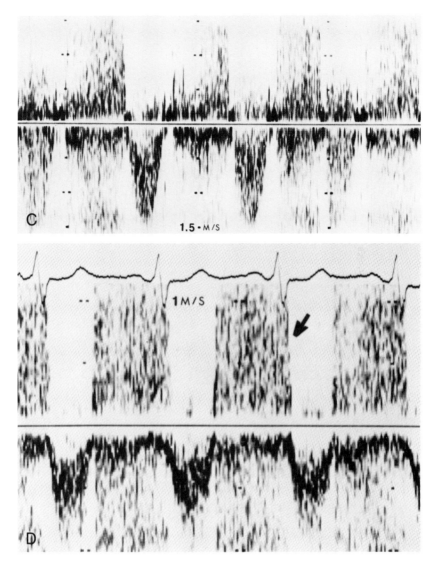

F<small>IGURE</small> 33 (continued).

diastolic blow was also appreciated. A_2 was well preserved. Carotid upstroke appeared somewhat diminished.

ECHOCARDIOGRAPHY AND DOPPLER FINDINGS

M-mode and 2-dimensional echocardiography revealed a calcified aortic root and valve and normal left ventricular function. Continuous-wave Doppler from the cardiac apex is shown in Figure 34A. A pulsed-Doppler tracing obtained from the LVOT 1.5 cm from the valve plane is shown in Figure 34B. A continuous-wave recording from the right parasternal region is shown in Figure 34C.

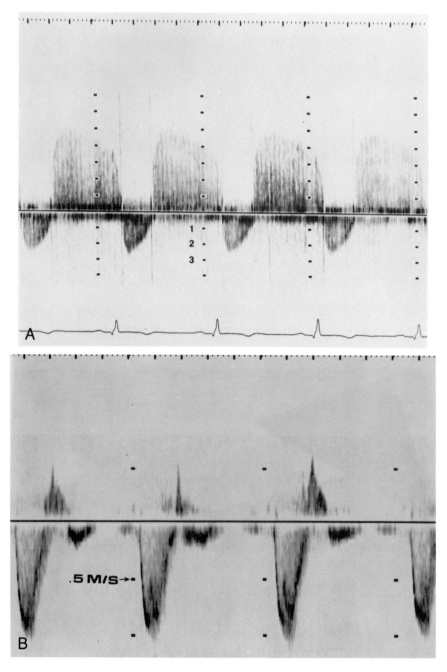

FIGURE 34.

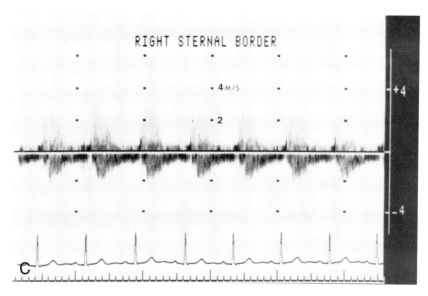

RIGHT STERNAL BORDER

FIGURE 34 (continued).

What is the diagnosis? _____

How significant are these lesions? _____

ANSWER

Continuous-wave recordings from the cardiac apex and the right parasternal regions reveal peak velocities of 2.9 m/sec. In the presence of normal left ventricular function, a transvalvular gradient of 33 mm Hg represents a mild to moderate degree of aortic stenosis. The aortic insufficiency seen in the continuous-wave recording maps back into the ventricle for only 1 cm above the valve plane. In addition, the slope of velocity decay seen on the continuous-wave tracing is relatively flat, supporting the diagnosis of mild aortic insufficiency. The patient was cleared for surgery and had an uneventful postoperative course.

Case #4

HISTORY AND PHYSICAL EXAMINATION

A 51-year-old man was admitted to the hospital for evaluation of exertional chest pain of three-months duration. Additional complaints included easy fatigability and dyspnea on moderate exertion. On physical examination, the left ventricular impulse was felt to be diminished, and a Grade III/VI systolic ejection murmur was heard in the aortic area without significant radiation.

ECHOCARDIOGRAPHY AND DOPPLER FINDINGS

M-mode and 2-dimensional echocardiography showed the left ventricle to be enlarged and mildly hypokinetic. There was diastolic flut-

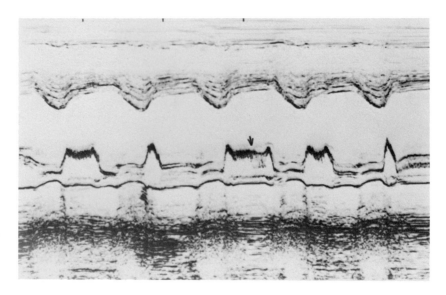

F<small>IGURE</small> 35.

tering of the anterior mitral leaflet (Figure 35). The aortic valve was bicuspid. Peak aortic velocity seen by continuous-wave Doppler from the cardiac apex is shown in Figure 36A, and that obtained from the suprasternal notch is shown in Figure 36B. LVOT velocity in pulsed Doppler measured 1.0 m/sec. The cross-sectional area of the aortic valve anulus was 4.4 cm².

What is the diagnosis? _____

What is the peak aortic valve gradient? _____

Calculate the aortic valve area. _____

ANSWER

This patient had aortic stenosis and insufficiency (arrows, Figures 35, 36). Peak velocities of 5 m/sec, measured from both the cardiac apex and parasternal windows, indicated a transvalvular peak aortic gradient of 100 mm Hg. Peak velocity measured from the suprasternal notch was approximately 4 m/sec. The patient underwent cardiac catheterization, at which time a peak systolic transvalvular gradient of 90 mm Hg was measured. The aortic valve area was severely reduced (0.7 cm²) in the presence of low cardiac output. Aortic valve area can be calculated by the equation:

$$AVA = \frac{V_{LVOT}}{V_{max}} \times CSA = \frac{1}{5} \times 4.4 = 0.9 \text{ cm}^2$$

References

Berger, M., Berdoff, R.L., Gallerstein, P.E., and Goldberg, E.: Evaluation of aortic stenosis by continuous wave Doppler ultrasound. J. Am. Coll. Cardiol., *3*:150–156, 1984.

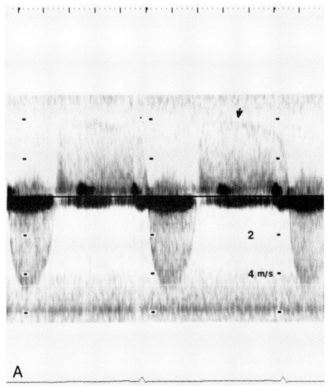

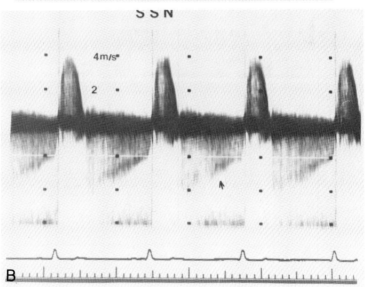

FIGURE 36.

Boughner, D.K.: Circulation, *52*:874–879, 1975.

Bryg, R.J., Pearson, A.C., Williams, G.A., and Labovitz, A.J.: Left ventricular systolic and diastolic flow abnormalities in hypertrophic obstructive cardiomyopathy. Am. J. Cardiol., *59*:925–931, 1987.

Ciobanu, M., Abbasi, A., Allen, M., Hermer, A., and Spellberg, R.: Pulsed Doppler echocardiography in the diagnosis and estimation of severity of aortic insufficiency. Am. J. Cardiol., *49*:339–343, 1982.

Currie, P.J., Seward, J.B., Reeder, G.S., Vlietstra, R.E., Bresnahan, D.R., Bresnahan, J.F., Smith, H.C., Hagler, D.J., and Tajik, A.J.: Continuous-wave Doppler echocardiographic assessment of severity of calcific aortic stenosis: A simultaneous Doppler-catheter correlative study in 100 adult patients. Circulation, *71*:1162–1169, 1985.

Goldberg, S.J. and Allen, M.: Quantitative assessment by Doppler echocardiography of pulmonary or aortic regurgitation. Am. J. Cardiol., *56*:131–135, 1985.

Hatle, L.: Noninvasive assessment and differentiation of left ventricular outflow obstruction with Doppler ultrasound. Circulation, *64*:380–387, 1981.

Kitabatake, A., Ito, H., Inoue, M., et al.: A new approach to noninvasive evaluation of aortic regurgitant fraction by two-dimensional Doppler echocardiography. Circulation, *72*:523–529, 1985.

Labovitz, A.J., Ferrara, R.P., Kern, M.J., Bryg, R.J., Mrosek, D.G., and Williams, G.A.: Quantitative evaluation of aortic insufficiency by continuous wave Doppler echocardiography. J. Am. Coll. Cardiol., *3*:1341–1347, 1986.

Quinones, M., Young, J.B., Waggoner, A.D., Ostojic, M.C., Ribeiro, L.G., and Miller, R.L.: Assessment of pulsed Doppler echocardiography in detection and quantitation of aortic and mitral regurgitation. Br. Heart. J., *44*:612–620, 1980.

Requarth, J.A., Goldberg, S.J., Vasko, S.D., and Allen, H.D.: In vitro verification of Doppler prediction of transvalve pressure gradient and orifice area in stenosis. Am. J. Cardiol., *53*:1369–1373, 1984.

Skjaerpe, T., Hergrenaes, L., and Hatle, L.: Noninvasive estimation of valve area in patients with aortic stenosis by Doppler ultrasound and two-dimensional echocardiography. Circulation, *72*:810–818, 1985.

Stamm, R.B., and Martin, R.P.: Quantitation of pressure gradients across stenotic valves by Doppler ultrasound. J. Am. Coll. Cardiol., *2*:707–718, 1983.

Teirstein, P., Yeager, M., Yock, P.G., and Popp, R.L.: Doppler echocardiographic measurement of aortic valve area in aortic stenosis: A noninvasive application of the Gorlin formula. J. Am. Coll. Cardiol., *8*:1059–1065, 1986.

Veyrat, C., Lessana, A., Abitbol, G., Ameur, A., Benaim, R. and Kalmanson, D.: New indexes for assessing aortic regurgitation with 2-dimensional Doppler echocardiographic measurement of the regurgitant aortic valvular area. Circulation, *68*:998–1005, 1983.

Williams, G.A., Labovitz, A.J., Nelson, J.G., and Kennedy, H.L.: Value of multiple echocardiographic views in the evaluation of aortic stenosis in adults by continuous wave Doppler. Am. J. Cardiol., *55*:445–449, 1985.

Worth, D.C., Stewart, W.J., Block, P.C., and Weyman, A.E.: A new method to calculate aortic valve area without left heart catheterization. Circulation, *70*:978–983, 1984.

Yock, P.G., Hatle, L., and Popp, R.L.: Patterns and timing of Doppler-detected intracavitary and aortic flow in hypertrophic cardiomyopathy. J. Am. Coll. Cardiol., *8*:1047–1058, 1986.

5

Mitral Valve Pathology

Mitral Stenosis

Doppler helps to evaluate the severity of mitral stenosis by both estimating the orifice area and giving some idea about pressures within the heart. A Doppler tracing of a normal mitral valve (Figure 37A) shows the following characteristics:

a maximum velocity about 1 m/sec
rapid deceleration of blood velocity after early diastolic filling.

In contrast, a Doppler tracing of a stenosed mitral valve (Figure 37B) reveals:

a maximum velocity greater than 1 m/sec
slower deceleration of blood velocity after early diastolic filling.

A stenotic mitral valve causes a pressure gradient between the left atrium and left ventricle, which becomes less as blood begins to flow from one chamber to the other. The pressure gradient is proportional to the orifice size and to the flow across the mitral valve. Rises in left atrial pressure occur with tachycardia or the demand for higher cardiac output. Doppler tracings of mitral stenosis reflect the hemodynamic changes as:

higher than normal velocities
slower decay of velocities (flat "E-F" slope), reflecting prolonged pressure gradients across the valve.

The severity of mitral valve disease can be estimated from the calculated size of the mitral valve orifice or the mean pressure gradient across the valve. Both give physiologic information helpful in the management of patients.

The mitral valve area is calculated by the pressure halftime method (see Chapter 3) (Figure 38). One must remember to: 1) use the actual outline of the "E-F" slope from the mitral valve Doppler tracing, 2) ignore the "A wave" if the patient is in sinus rhythm, 3) use paper

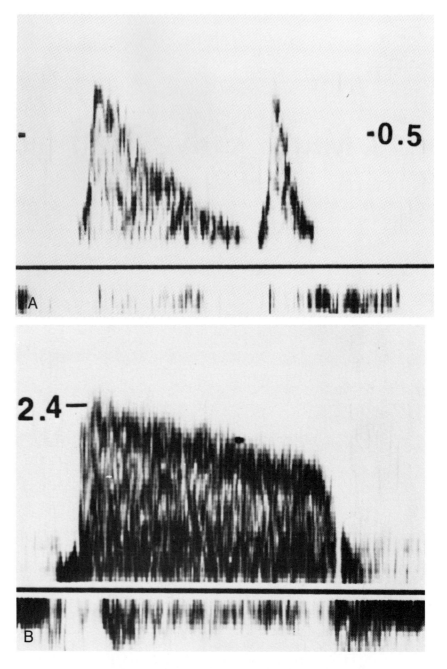

FIGURE 37.   Normal mitral valve flow (A). Peak velocity is less than 1.0 m/sec, and velocity decays rapidly until atrial flow increases. Mitral stenosis (B). Peak velocity is higher than normal, and velocity decays gradually through diastole.

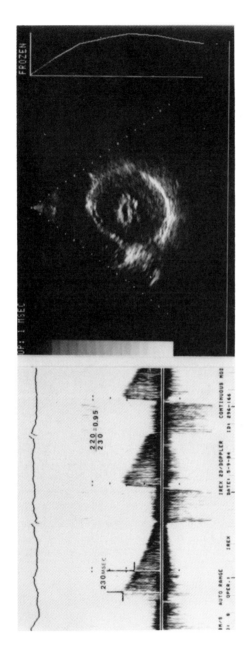

FIGURE 38.   Calculation of mitral valve area. 2D echo (right) shows a narrowed, calcified mitral valve. Doppler (left) shows the typical slow diastolic decay of velocity. The pressure halftime method is demonstrated.

speeds of 50–100 mm/sec because the apparent pressure halftime can vary slightly due to measurement errors, and 4) average 3–5 beats if the patient is in sinus rhythm and 5–10 beats if atrial fibrillation is present.

To calculate the mean mitral valve pressure gradient, divide the diastolic flow into five to nine equally spaced segments, square each velocity, and then use the average of the squares of the velocities in the calculation (Figure 39). One can test the physiologic effects of the stenosis by calculating the gradient at rest and then again after the patient has exercised and has a raised heart rate.

Recordings are best made from the apex (Figure 40). Initial scanning with Doppler should be done in the continuous mode to locate the highest velocities, to look for mitral regurgitation, and to best align the interrogating beam with the stenotic jet (Figure 41). Pulsed or high-PRF modes can then be used to improve the clarity of the spectral tracing.

Mitral Regurgitation

Mitral regurgitation is displayed by Doppler as systolic velocities of 2 m/sec or greater across the mitral valve from left ventricle to left atrium. Although systolic jets can be recorded, the calculated pressure gradient has not proven useful for predicting left atrial pressures.

Scanning for the presence of mitral regurgitation is best done from the apical view using continuous-wave Doppler. Since the regurgitant blood flow jet can occur at any angle, the whole left atrium should be interrogated.

Pulsed-Flow Mapping

Once the high velocity jet of mitral regurgitation has been found (Figure 42), it can be mapped back into the left atrium using pulsed-mode Doppler (Figure 43). Starting at the valve plane, the Doppler sample volume is moved progressively deeper into the left atrium until a systolic flow disturbance is no longer seen or heard. Mitral regurgitant jets can occur at any angle to the valve, and may not be adequately followed in the plane of the four-chamber view. In addition, the enlarged heart may displace the atrium to too great a depth to be adequately sampled in the four-chamber view. For these reasons, both the four-chamber and long-axis (apical or parasternal) views should be used when "mapping" a regurgitant jet.

Regurgitation can be qualitatively graded by observation. With mild mitral regurgitation, flow is seen only at the valve plane; with moderate mitral regurgitation, the flow extends to the mid left atrium; and with severe mitral regurgitation, flow can be mapped into the distal portion of the left atrium.

A simplified quantitative method is to define mild mitral regurgita-

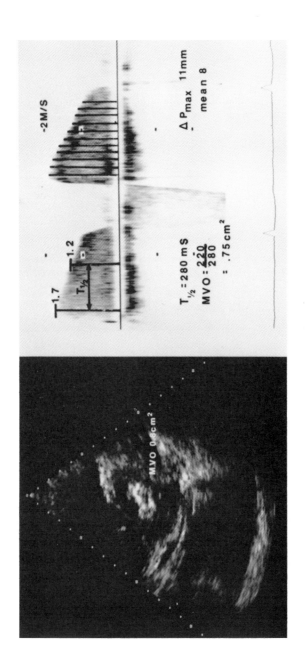

FIGURE 39. Calculation of orifice area and gradient. The anatomic orifice (left) has an area of 0.8 cm². Calculation by the pressure halftime method using Doppler velocities (right) gives a similar result. Although the peak pressure is 11 mm Hg, the mean pressure drop is 8 mm Hg.

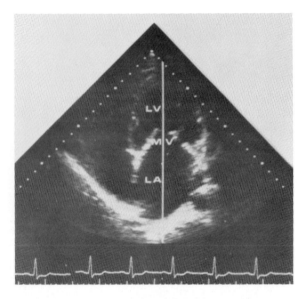

FIGURE 40. Two-dimensional image showing displacement of the transducer laterally to align the interrogating beam more accurately with presumed mitral flow. Often, the best recording of velocity is obtained with the transducer cursor positioned in the apparent orifice, but slightly off center.

tion as a flow disturbance extending less than 2 cm into the left atrium, and moderate to severe mitral regurgitation as a flow disturbance extending more than 2 cm into the left atrium.

Newer Methods

Recent reports have shown that calculation of the mitral regurgitant fraction (see Chapter 8) may be useful in assessing the degree of mitral insufficiency. Color flow Doppler has also been used to determine the degree of insufficiency (Figure 44).

Combined Mitral Valve Disease

Rheumatic mitral valve disease often presents as a mixed lesion, i.e., a combination of stenosis and regurgitation. In addition, rhythm abnormalities, especially atrial fibrillation, are common. A recent study comparing the pressure halftime method to two-dimensional echocardiography has shown that Doppler remains reliable for calculating mitral valve area under these conditions.

Mitral Anular Calcification

Mitral anular calcification is a frequent echocardiographic finding in elderly persons, in whom heart murmurs and other nonspecific signs

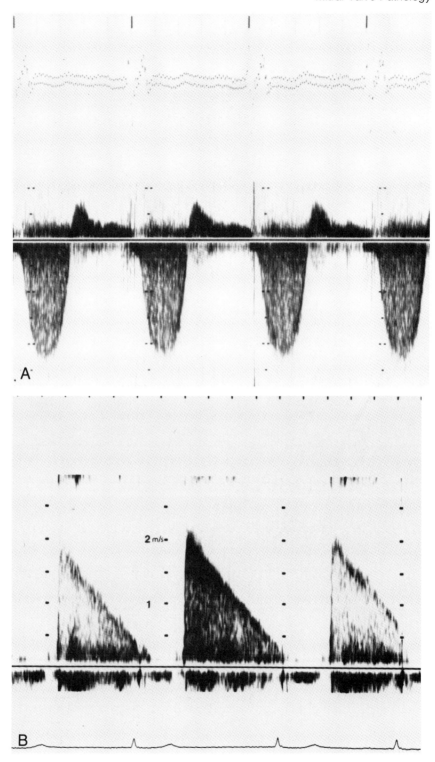

FIGURE 41.   Continuous-wave tracing of combined mitral stenosis and regurgitation (A). High systolic velocities oriented away from the transducer confirm the presence of an insufficient jet. (B) Well-aligned tracing of the jet of mitral stenosis. Velocity profile is well outlined, and high velocity reflectors produce the highest intensity (darkest portion of the tracing).

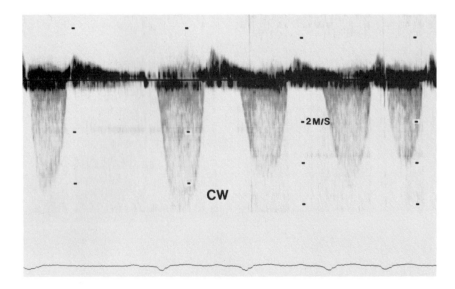

FIGURE 42. Continuous-wave tracing from a patient with mitral regurgitation. Note variation in maximal velocity due to changes in diastolic filling time: velocities are higher after long cycles, reflecting higher intraventricular pressure.

and symptoms suggest hemodynamically significant lesions. Doppler evaluation of transmitral flow is useful in the diagnosis of functional mitral stenosis, as well as mitral regurgitation, in individuals not sufficiently symptomatic to warrant cardiac catheterization.

Mitral Valve Pathology Case Studies

Case #1

HISTORY AND PHYSICAL EXAMINATION

The patient is a 47-year-old female who developed breathlessness on climbing stairs. She had rheumatic fever as a child but was felt to have recovered. Two pregnancies were completed normally.

On examination, she had an accentuated first heart sound. Her second heart sound was loud at the apex. An opening snap was heard at the apex. No murmurs were present.

Pulsed-wave Doppler of the mitral valve flow is shown in Figure 45.

What is the maximum velocity? _____

What is the pressure halftime? _____

What is the mitral valve orifice area? _____

ANSWER

This patient represents a case of mild mitral stenosis. The mitral valve velocity is increased to 2.2 m/sec. The diastolic decay is rapid and the pressure halftime is 100 msec, indicating a valve area of 2.2

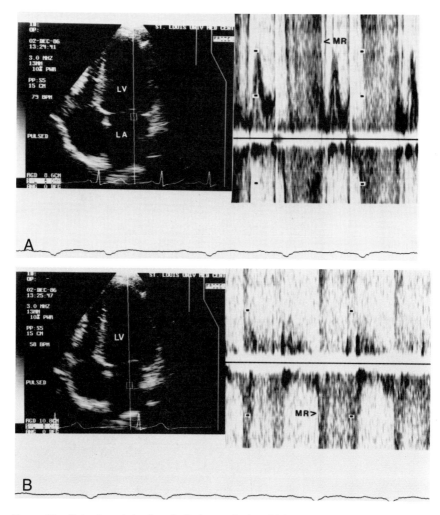

FIGURE 43.   Pulsed-mode tracing of mitral regurgitation. (A) Sample volume has been moved to the point where regurgitant velocities (arrow, MR) are first identified. (B) Sample volume has been positioned at the deepest level where regurgitant velocities are seen.

cm^2. However, the patient's resting heart rate is 80, and the mean trans-valvular gradient is elevated to 11 mm Hg. With higher heart rates, the mean gradient and left atrial pressure would be expected to rise further, explaining her dyspnea.

Case #2

HISTORY AND PHYSICAL EXAMINATION

A 65-year-old female had been treated for atrial fibrillation for several years and was recovering from surgery for removal of a femoral embolus, questionably of cardiac origin.

Physical examination revealed an irregular rhythm, a loud first heart sound, a systolic ejection murmur at the right upper sternal border, and

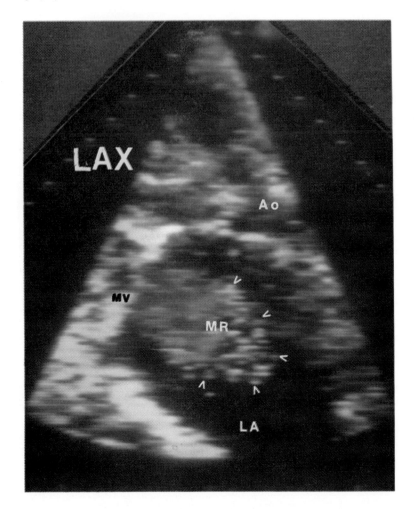

FIGURE 44. Mitral insufficiency, color Doppler in the long-axis view (LAX). Regurgitant jet (MR) is clearly seen (arrows) in the left atrium (LA) during systole.

a loud P_2. A soft opening snap and early diastolic rumble were present at the cardiac apex.

Two-dimensional echocardiography revealed mitral stenosis with a pliable mitral valve, left atrial enlargement, and an atrial thrombus. Her Doppler is shown in Figure 46.

Does the Doppler add to the physical findings? _____

What is the pressure halftime? _____

What is the mitral orifice area? _____

ANSWER

This patient demonstrates many of the findings characteristic of moderately severe mitral stenosis. Her pressure halftime varies slightly from beat to beat (160–190 msec), averaging 170 msec. The calculated valve area is 1.3 cm², consistent with moderately severe mitral stenosis. Due

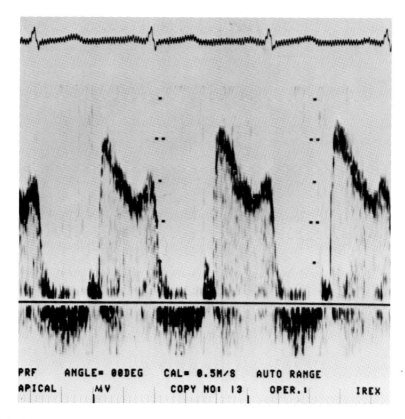

F<small>IGURE</small> 45.

to the presence of atrial fibrillation and a slow heart rate, however, her mean transmitral gradient is low and approaches zero during long dia-stolic intervals (beat 4). Thus, this patient did well clinically until the thromboembolism.

When evaluating patients with atrial fibrillation, it is important to use multiple cycles and to follow the actual velocity tracing. While velocity in the first and second beats decays along a straight line, the profile of the third and fourth beats is slightly curved. Trying to estimate the pressure halftime by a line drawn with a ruler could underestimate or overestimate the actual halftime. In Figure 47, a line drawn along the steepest portion of the curve (line A) would overestimate the orifice area. A line from the peak to the end of curve (B) would underestimate it by artifactually prolonging pressure halftime. The actual pressure halftime velocity (point C) lies between the points defined by the two lines.

Case #3

HISTORY AND PHYSICAL EXAMINATION

A 64-year-old man presented with progressive heart failure and edema. He had had rheumatic heart disease and was being evaluated for aortic valve surgery.

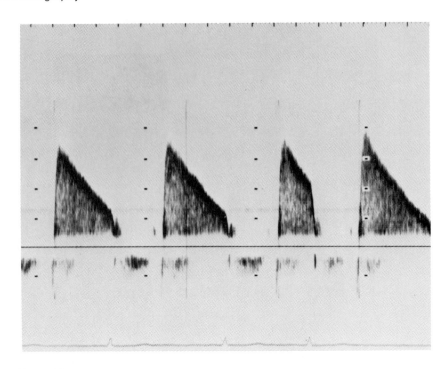

FIGURE 46.

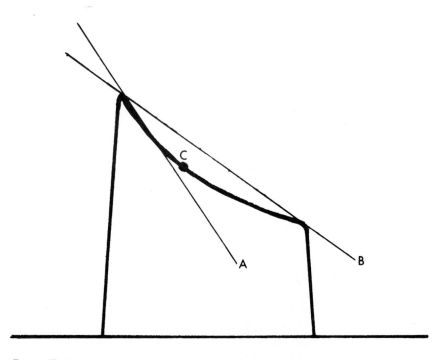

FIGURE 47.

On echocardiography, his mitral valve was found to be calcified and no orifice area could be measured. He had borderline low left ventricular function. Figure 48 shows a continuous-wave Doppler tracing of the mitral (A) and aortic (B) valves.

What is the peak aortic gradient? _____

What is the maximal mitral velocity? _____

What is the pressure halftime velocity? _____

What is the pressure halftime? _____

What is the mitral orifice area? _____

ANSWER

The maximal aortic velocity is approximately 3.6 m/sec, calculating to a 52-mm Hg aortic valve gradient. As was seen in the aortic valve section (Chapter 4), this may represent severe stenosis when left ventricular dysfunction is present. The patient also has aortic insufficiency, which by the pattern and mapping remains mild.

Maximum mitral velocity = 2.5 m/sec, pressure halftime velocity = 1.8 m/sec, pressure halftime (average) = 250 msec, calculated mitral valve area = 0.9 cm².

When evaluating for rheumatic heart disease, it is important to interrogate both mitral and aortic valves. Aortic insufficiency can cause

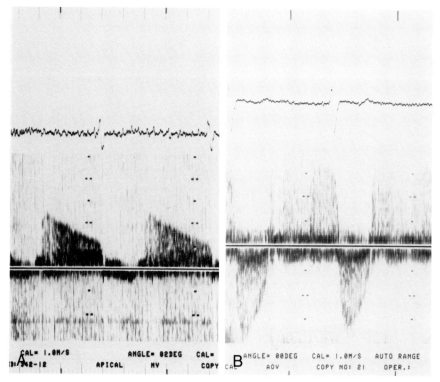

FIGURE 48.

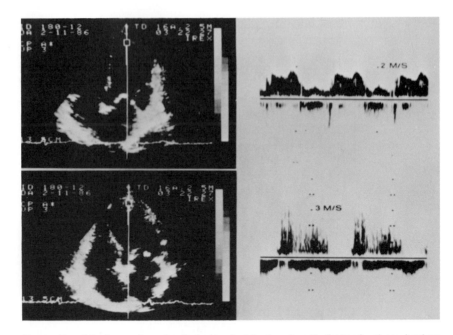

FIGURE 49. Apical recording of pathologic mitral (top) and aortic (bottom) valves. A minor shift in transducer angulation moves the inquiring beam out of the mitral stenosis jet and into the aortic insufficiency flow, making it important to record velocities from both valves when one is diseased.

either underestimation or overestimation of the mitral valve orifice area. If the aortic valve is not interrogated properly, the jet of aortic insufficiency can be mistaken for that of a stenotic mitral valve (Figure 49). Calculations using the aortic insufficiency tracing can seriously underestimate the mitral valve orifice area.

The pressure halftime method relies on changes in left atrial and ventricular pressure due to flow across the mitral valve. In aortic insufficiency, left ventricular pressure rises due to the filling of the left ventricle from both the left atrium and the aorta. Due to competing flow from the aorta, left ventricular pressure rises faster than normally, and the mitral pressure halftime may be shortened in decompensated aortic insufficiency. In patients with compensated aortic insufficiency, the halftime relation is preserved. It is important, therefore, to scan both mitral and aortic valves.

Case #4

HISTORY AND PHYSICAL EXAMINATION

A 46-year-old male with Marfan's syndrome presented with gradually worsening dyspnea on exertion. On examination, he had a late systolic murmur obscuring his other heart sounds.

Figure 50A shows the M-mode and continuous-wave Doppler tracings obtained at the examination. Figure 50B shows the pulsed-mode tracing obtained approximately 2 cm into the left atrium.

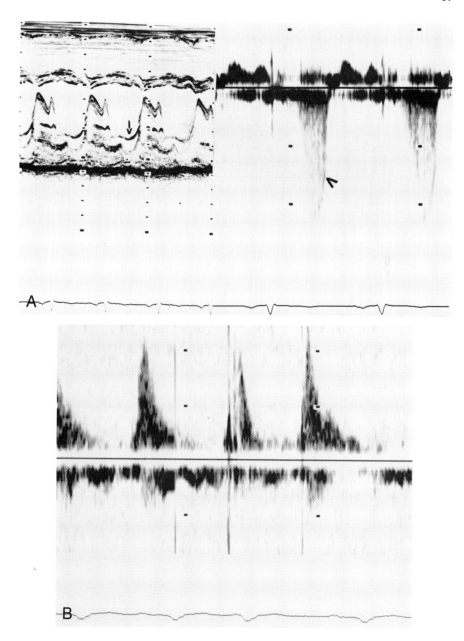

F<small>IGURE</small> 50.

What is the anatomic diagnosis? _____

What is the physiologic abnormality? _____

Is mitral stenosis present? _____

ANSWER

  The continuous-wave tracing (Figure 50A) reveals late systolic flow
away from the transducer, compatible with mitral regurgitation. The

pulsed mode shows only diastolic velocities, indicating mild mitral insufficiency.

References

Abbasi, A.S., Allen, M.W., DeCristofaro, D., and Ungar, I.: Detection and estimation of the degree of mitral regurgitation by pulsed Doppler echocardiography. Circulation, *61*:143–147, 1980.

Ascah, K.J., Stewart, W.J., Jiang, L., Guerrero, J.L., Newell, J.B., Gillam, L.D., and Weyman, A.E.: A Doppler two-dimensional echocardiographic method for quantitation of mitral regurgitation. Circulation, *72*:377–383, 1985.

Blanchard, D., Diebold, B., Peronneau, P., Foult, J.M., Nee, M., Guermonprez, J.L., and Maurice, P.: Non-invasive diagnosis of mitral regurgitation by Doppler echocardiography. Br. Heart J., *45*:589–593, 1981.

Blumlein, S., Bouchard, A., Schiller, N.B., Dae, M., Byrd, B.F., Ports, T., and Botvinick, E.H.: Quantitation of mitral regurgitation by Doppler echocardiography. Circulation, *74*:306–314, 1986.

Bryg, R.J., Williams, G.A., Labovitz, A.J., Aker, U., and Kennedy, H.L.: Effect of atrial fibrillation and mitral regurgitation on calculated mitral valve area in mitral stenosis. Am. J. Cardiol., *57*:634–638, 1986.

Erzengin, F., and Williams, G.: An evaluation of aortic and mitral regurgitation by pulsed Doppler echocardiography compared to angiography. Eur. Heart J., *5*:10, 1984.

Hatle, L., Angelsen, B., and Tromsdal, A.: Non-invasive assessment of atrioventricular pressure halftime by Doppler ultrasound. Circulation, *69*:1096–1104, 1969.

Labovitz, A.J., Nelson, J.G., Windhorst, D.M., Kennedy, H.L., and Williams, G.A.: Frequency of mitral valve dysfunction from mitral annular calcium as detected by Doppler echocardiography. Am. J. Cardiol., *55*:133–137, 1985.

Miyatake, K., Izumi, S., Okamoto, M., Kinoshita, N., Asonuma, H., Nakagawa, H., Yamamoto, K., Takamiya, M., Sakakibara, H., and Nimura, Y.: Semiquantitative grading of severity of mitral regurgitation by real-time two-dimensional Doppler flow imaging technique. J. Am. Coll. Cardiol., *7*:82–88, 1986.

Miyatake, K., Kinoshita, N., Nagata, S., Beppu, S., Park, Y.D.; Sakakibara, H., and Nimura, Y.: Intracardiac flow pattern in mitral regurgitation studied with combined use of the ultrasonic pulsed Doppler technique and cross-sectional echocardiography. Am. J. Cardiol., *45*:155–162, 1980.

Quinones, M., Young, J.B., Waggoner, A.D., Ostojic, M.C., Ribeiro, L.G., and Miller, R.L.: Assessment of pulsed Doppler echocardiography in detection and quantitation of aortic and mitral regurgitation. Br. Heart J., *44*:612–620, 1980.

Stamm, R.B., and Martin, R.P.: Quantitation of pressure gradients across stenotic valves by Doppler ultrasound. J. Am. Coll. Cardiol., *2*:707–718, 1983.

6

Right Heart Valves

Tricuspid Valve Pathology

The tricuspid valve lies in the same plane as the mitral valve, and can be evaluated from the cardiac apex. The Doppler beam should be directed parallel to the blood flow from the right atrium into the right ventricle (Figure 51).

Due to the right ventricle's unusual anatomy, the tricuspid valve can also be interrogated from the left parasternal area. The transducer is oriented for a short-axis view of the aorta and aimed inferiorly, or moved one interspace lower to orient the beam correctly for the tricuspid flow.

The most common tricuspid valve disease is tricuspid insufficiency. High velocity regurgitant jets can be recorded in systole from the right ventricle to the right atrium (Figure 52) and can be quantitated to provide valuable information.

Calculation of a systolic pressure gradient across the tricuspid valve, using the regurgitant velocity and the Bernoulli equation ($P_1 - P_2 = 4V^2$), gives an accurate estimate of the systolic pressure difference between the right ventricle and right atrium. Adding the estimated right atrial pressure to the calculated gradient then gives an estimate of right ventricular and pulmonary systolic pressure.

In the presence of tricuspid regurgitation and normal pulmonary artery pressures, calculated gradients across the tricuspid valve are less than 25 mm Hg (a maximum velocity of 2.5 m/sec), but gradients and velocities may be greater if pulmonary hypertension is present. Thus, one can tell if tricuspid regurgitation is due to a diseased tricuspid valve with normal pulmonary pressure or secondary to pulmonary hypertension.

Regurgitant-flow-mapping techniques can also be used in the right atrium. Tricuspid insufficiency can be graded as mild (within 1 cm of the valve), moderate (1–3 cm into the right atrium), or severe (greater than 3 cm into the right atrium). Tricuspid stenosis occurs in approximately 5% of patients with rheumatic heart disease and is characterized by Doppler as increased velocities and decreased pressures half-time (Figure 53).

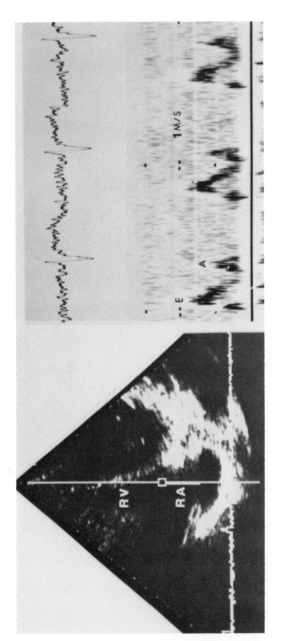

FIGURE 51.   Tricuspid valve flow recorded from the apical window.

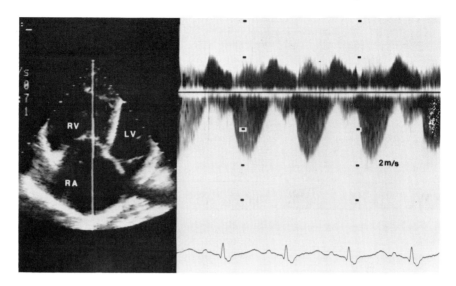

FIGURE 52. Tricuspid insufficiency. Regurgitant flow velocities are seen in systole and can be used to predict right ventricular pressures.

Pulmonic Valve Pathology

The pulmonic valve is approached from the short axis of the aorta by angulation of the transducer superiorly and to the patient's left.

Pulmonary valve stenosis is rare except in pediatric age groups. Doppler estimates of pulmonic stenosis gradients have been shown to be diagnostic and accurate.

The evaluation of pulmonary insufficiency is more difficult. Doppler

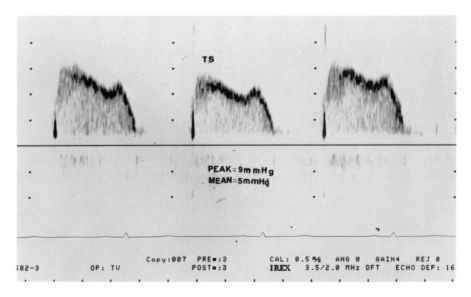

FIGURE 53. Tricuspid stenosis. Diastolic velocities are elevated, and the calculated mean pressure gradient is 5 mm Hg, suggesting significant stenosis.

is extremely sensitive for insufficiency, and both minimal tricuspid and pulmonic insufficiency can be seen in normals. Continuous-mode Doppler in the pulmonary artery may also detect nearby coronary flow. Therefore, pulmonary insufficiency should be considered only if there is a flow disturbance in the right ventricular outflow tract below the pulmonic valve in the pulsed mode, and should be considered abnormal only if it extends more than 1 cm into the right ventricular outflow tract.

Evaluation of Pulmonary Pressures

Several methods have been reported for using Doppler ultrasound to estimate pulmonary artery pressures. Application of the modified Bernoulli equation to the maximal velocity found in the jet of individuals with tricuspid regurgitation provides an accurate estimate of pulmonary artery systolic pressure in the absence of valvular pulmonic stenosis. The vast majority of individuals with elevated pulmonary artery systolic pressure will in fact have Doppler-detectable tricuspid regurgitation, thus enabling the calculation of the pulmonary artery pressure. Several reports have also suggested analysis of the pulmonary artery velocity waveform to calculate mean pulmonary artery pressure. The ratio of acceleration time (from onset of flow to peak velocity) divided by the right ventricular ejection time is inversely proportional to the mean pulmonary artery pressure, i.e., the more rapidly the peak velocity is reached, the higher the mean pulmonary artery pressure (Figure 54). Finally, one recent report suggests that analysis of the end diastolic velocity in individuals with pulmonic insufficiency may provide a means to estimate pulmonary capillary wedge pressure.

Tricuspid Valve Pathology Case Studies

Case #1

HISTORY AND PHYSICAL EXAMINATION

A 24-year-old female was being evaluated for a heart murmur, present since her midteens. She was asymptomatic. Physical examination disclosed a systolic click and a mid-to-late systolic murmur at the cardiac apex.

She had mitral valve prolapse on 2-dimensional echocardiography. The echo was otherwise normal.

Figure 55 shows a continuous-wave recording of the tricuspid valve from the cardiac apex.

What is the diagnosis? _____

What is the peak systolic velocity? _____

What is the gradient? _____

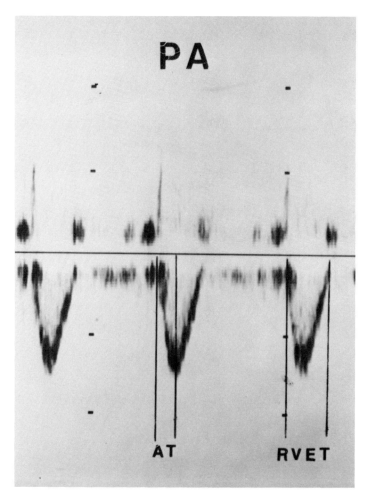

FIGURE 54. Pulmonary artery velocity profile. Acceleration time (AT) is the interval from onset of flow to peak velocity. Right ventricular ejection time (RVET) is the total time of flow.

ANSWER

Doppler is extremely sensitive and, in the continuous mode, will record all flow present within the interrogating beam. This patient did not have tricuspid insufficiency clinically, and her valve appeared normal by 2-dimensional echocardiography. The peak systolic velocity of 2.5 m/sec and calculated gradient of 25 mm Hg reflect normal right ventricular systolic pressure. It is common to find minimal tricuspid regurgitation by Doppler in patients with normal hemodynamics and anatomically normal tricuspid valves, possibly due to the tricuspid valve's larger area (5 to 8 cm^2) and trileaflet structure. In the final report, regurgitation may be noted as physiologic, insignificant, or not mentioned at all.

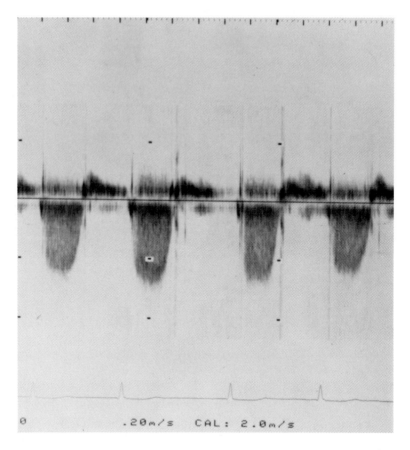

FIGURE 55.

Case #2

HISTORY AND PHYSICAL EXAMINATION

A 27-year-old female presented with a murmur persisting since birth. She had moderate dyspnea on exertion and limited herself to light housework. Examination revealed a Grade II/VI holosystolic and diastolic "machinery" murmur at the left upper sternal border, and a Grade IV systolic murmur at the left lower sternal border. Her liver was pulsatile, and large jugular V waves were observed. Echocardiograms confirmed right ventricular enlargement and volume overload. Continuous-wave Doppler of her tricuspid valve is shown in Figure 56 (vertical calibration marks indicate 2-m/sec steps).

What is the diagnosis? _____

What is the peak velocity? _____

What is the gradient? _____

ANSWER

The Doppler in this patient confirms the clinical diagnosis of tricuspid regurgitation. The peak velocity of 4 m/sec and calculated gradient

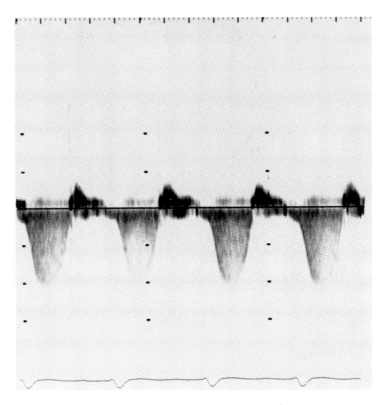

FIGURE 56.

of 64 mm Hg indicate severe pulmonary hypertension. The clinical finding of a machinery murmur along with the elevated pressure suggests congenital heart disease with a patent ductus arteriosus. Cardiac catheterization confirmed a patent ductus arteriosus and found a pulmonary artery systolic pressure of 70 mm Hg, similar to that calculated from the Doppler study.

Pulmonic Valve Pathology Case Studies

Case #1

HISTORY AND PHYSICAL EXAMINATION

A 12-year-old male was seen by his pediatrician for chest pain during soccer practice. He had a known systolic heart murmur at the left upper sternal border, but had felt well and had previously exhibited normal growth and activity.

The 2-dimensional echocardiography was non-diagnostic. The right ventricular size was at the upper limits of normal, and the pulmonary valve was not well visualized.

The continuous-wave Doppler spectral tracing in Figure 57 is of the pulmonary valve.

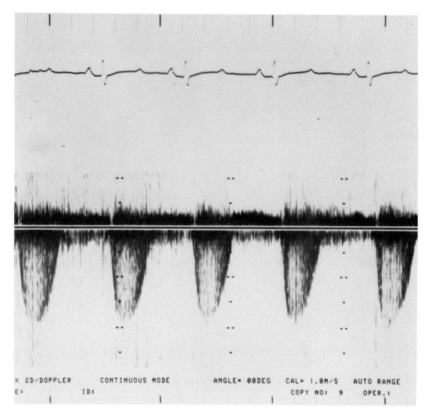

X 2D/DOPPLER   CONTINUOUS MODE   ANGLE= 00DEG   CAL= 1.0M/S   AUTO RANGE
E: ID: COPY NO: 9   OPER.:

FIGURE 57.

What is the Doppler diagnosis? ⎯⎯⎯⎯⎯⎯⎯⎯⎯⎯⎯⎯⎯⎯⎯⎯⎯⎯
What is the maximal velocity? ⎯⎯⎯⎯⎯⎯⎯⎯⎯⎯⎯⎯⎯⎯⎯⎯⎯⎯
What is the gradient? ⎯⎯⎯⎯⎯⎯⎯⎯⎯⎯⎯⎯⎯⎯⎯⎯⎯⎯⎯⎯⎯⎯⎯

ANSWER

This patient has the findings of pulmonic stenosis. The maximal velocity of 3.8 m/sec reflects a gradient of 58 mm Hg across the pulmonary valve. On this basis, the patient was sent to catheterization and surgery for a pulmonary valvotomy.

Case #2

HISTORY AND PHYSICAL EXAMINATION

A 53-year-old female had a pulmonary valvotomy at one year of age. She was asymptomatic and was being studied as part of a routine follow-up.

The 2-dimensional echocardiogram revealed mild right ventricular enlargement.

Figure 58 is a pulsed-mode tracing from the right ventricular outflow

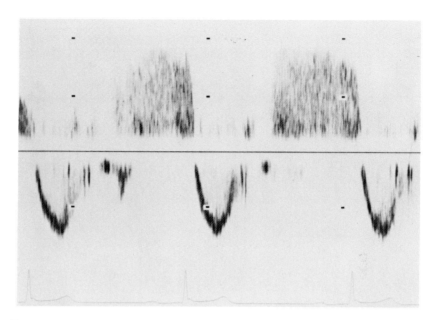

Figure 58.

tract. A continuous-wave tracing across the pulmonic valve revealed a peak velocity of approximately 2.7 m/sec.

What is the Doppler diagnosis? _____

Is the tracing diagnostic for insufficiency? _____

What is the pulmonary valve gradient from the peak velocity? _____

ANSWER

This case demonstrates mild residual pulmonic stenosis and insufficiency after repair of a stenotic pulmonary valve. The calculated systolic gradient from the maximal velocity (2.7 m/sec) is 29 mm Hg. The normal right ventricular outflow tract velocity (0.7 m/sec), seen within the systolic envelope in the continuous-wave and pulsed-mode tracings, does not contribute significantly to the Bernoulli equation.

The finding of a diastolic velocity on the continuous-wave tracing does not by itself make the diagnosis of pulmonic insufficiency definitive, since flow in coronary arteries may mimic pulmonic insufficiency in this view. However, the pulsed-mode tracing, with the sample volume in the right ventricular outflow tract, confirms that the diastolic velocities are caused by insufficient flow through the pulmonary valve.

References

Berger, M., Haimowitz, A., VanTosh, A., Berdoff, R.L., and Goldberg, E.: Quantitative assessment of pulmonary hypertension in patients with tricuspid regurgitation using continuous wave Doppler ultrasound. J. Am. Coll. Cardiol., *6*:359–365, 1985.

Currie, P.J., Seward, J.B., Chan, K.L., Fyfe, D.A., Hagler, D.J., Mair, D.D., Reeder, G.S., Nishimura, R.A., and Tajik, A.J.: Continuous wave Doppler determination of right ventricular pressure: A simultaneous Doppler-catheterization study in 127 patients. J. Am. Coll. Cardiol., *6*:75–76, 1985.

Dabestani, A., French, J., Gardin, J., Allfie, A., Russell, D., Burn, C., and Henry, W.: Doppler hepatic vein blood flow in patients with tricuspid regurgitation. Am. J. Cardiol., *1*:658, 1983.

Garcia-Dorado, D., Falzgraf, S., Almazan, A., Delcan, J.L., Lopez-Bescos, L., and Menarguez, L.: Diagnosis of functional tricuspid insufficiency by pulsed-wave Doppler ultrasound. Circulation, *66*:1315–1321, 1982.

Isobe, M., Yazaki, Y., Takaku, F., Koizumi, K., Hara, K., Tsuneyoski, H., Yamaguchi, T., and Machii, K.: Prediction of pulmonary arterial pressure in adults by pulsed Doppler echocardiography. Am. J. Cardiol., *57*:316–321, 1986.

Kitabatake, A., Inoue, M., Asao, M., Masuyama, T., Tanouchi, J., Morita, M., Uematsu, M., Shimazu, T., Hori, M., and Abe, H.: Noninvasive evaluation of pulmonary hypertension by a pulsed Doppler technique. Circulation, *68*:302–309, 1983.

Kosturakis, D., Goldberg, S.J., Allen, H.D., and Loeber, C.: Doppler echocardiographic prediction of pulmonary arterial hypertension in congenital heart disease. Am. J. Cardiol., *53*:1110–1115, 1984.

Masuyama, T., Kodama, K., Kitabatake, A., Sato, H., Nanto, S., and Inoue, M.: Continuous-wave Doppler echocardiographic detection of pulmonary regurgitation and its application to noninvasive estimation of pulmonary artery pressure. Circulation, *74*:484–492, 1986.

Miyatake, K., Okamoto, M., Kinoshita, N., Ohta, M., Kozuka, T., Sakakibara, H., and Nimura, Y.: Evaluation of tricuspid regurgitation by pulsed Doppler and 2-dimensional echocardiography. Circulation, *66*:777–784, 1982.

Suzuki, Y., Kambara, H., Kadota, K., Tamaki, S., Yamazato, A., Nohara, R., Osakada, G., and Kawai, C.: Detection and evaluation of tricuspid regurgitation using a real-time, two-dimensional, color-coded, Doppler flow imaging system: Comparison with contrast two-dimensional echocardiography and right ventriculography. Am. J. Cardiol., *57*:811–815, 1986.

Veyrat, C., Kalmanson, D., Farjon, M., Manin, J.P., and Abitol, G.: Non-invasive diagnosis and assessment of tricuspid regurgitation and stenosis using one and 2-dimensional echo-pulsed Doppler. Br. Heart J., *47*:596–605, 1982.

Yock, P., and Popp, R.: Non-invasive measurement of right ventricular systolic pressure by Doppler ultrasound in patients with tricuspid regurgitation. Circulation, *70*:657–662, 1984.

7

Prosthetic Valves

Prior to the advent of Doppler techniques, the noninvasive evaluation of prosthetic valves was limited. X-ray or echocardiographic visualization could sometimes identify dehiscence or masses, but the large majority of malfunctioning prostheses required cardiac catheterization for confirmation.

Prosthetic heart valves may be mechanical (ball-in-cage or disc) or made from tissue (usually porcine aortic valves). Mechanical valves are thrombogenic, and clots can cause obstruction of the orifice, insufficiency by preventing valve closure, or emboli. Tissue valves are less subject to thrombosis, but may be infected or degenerate, causing leakage or stenosis. All types of prosthetic valves may tear loose from the valve anulus (dehisce).

Evaluating prosthetic valves by Doppler is similar to evaluating native valves. The mitral valve is interrogated from the apex of the left ventricle and left parasternal window, and the aortic valve from three windows: apex, right parasternal area, and suprasternal notch.

Mitral

Prosthetic mitral valves all offer some obstruction to flow, which resembles mild mitral stenosis on a Doppler tracing. The pressure half-time method can then be used to calculate the effective orifice area. The following table summarizes Doppler findings in normally functioning prosthetic mitral valves:

Type	Valve Area		Mild Insufficiency
	Mean	Range	
Bjork-Shiley	2.4	1.6–3.7	25%
St. Jude	2.8	1.8–5.0	30%
Porcine	2.2	1.1–4.0	30%
Starr-Edwards	2.1	1.2–2.5	20%
Beall	1.7	1.3–2.0	—

Similar results have been reported for Medtronic disc valves. Care must be taken to interrogate the entire prosthesis for the best Doppler profile.

While disc and tissue valves are relatively easy to interrogate, Starr-Edwards valves must be carefully investigated to record flow around the occluder ball. The effective valve orifice area in normally functioning prosthetic mitral valves may vary with blood flow and valve size. A baseline study is therefore useful for all prosthetic valves for later comparison.

Evaluation for prosthetic mitral regurgitation requires careful examination of the left atrium from both the apex and left parasternal areas. Mild mitral regurgitation may be seen in normally functioning prosthetic valves, but moderate-to-severe mitral regurgitation is always abnormal.

Aortic

Prosthetic aortic valves have hemodynamics similar to mild aortic stenosis because their orifices are smaller than those of native valves. Doppler interrogation of prosthetic aortic valves reveals mild systolic gradients that can be calculated with the modified Bernoulli equation:

$$Gradient = 4 \ V^2_{max}$$

The following table summarizes Doppler findings for normally functioning prosthetic aortic valves:

Type	Calculated Gradient, mm Hg		Mild Insufficiency
	Peak	*Range*	
Bjork-Shiley	25	5–38	55%
St. Jude	22	4–38	58%
Starr-Edwards	36	12–50	55%
Porcine	26	4–36	40%

Similar results have been reported for Medtronic disc valves.

In general, all but the smallest aortic valves have Doppler peak gradients less than 40 mm Hg. Starr-Edwards valves in small sizes have gradients up to 50 mm Hg.

Mild aortic insufficiency by Doppler is a common finding in prosthetic aortic valves, but moderate-to-severe aortic insufficiency is usually pathologic.

Individual variability will be seen by Doppler in patients with normally functioning prosthetic valves secondary to valve size and position as well as left ventricular function. For this reason, a baseline Doppler evaluation is advisable in order to aid in the future diagnosis of valve malfunction.

Color flow Doppler has recently been reported to be useful in the evaluation of prosthetic valves (Figure 59), especially in patients with suspected paravalvular leak.

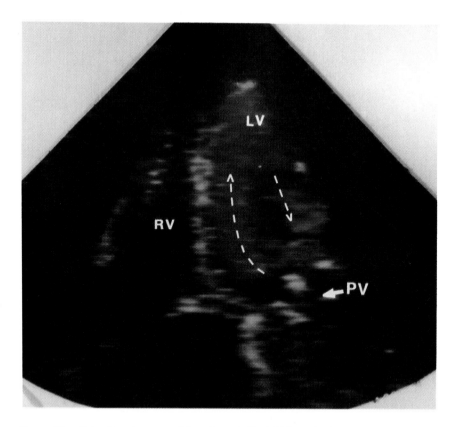

FIGURE 59. Color Doppler scan of flow through Bjork-Shiley mitral valve prosthesis (PV). Note the orientation of flow through the disc with vortex formation (dashed arrows).

Prosthetic Valve Pathology Case Studies

Case #1

HISTORY AND PHYSICAL EXAMINATION

A 32-year-old male was admitted to the hospital for evaluation of moderately severe congestive heart failure. Dyspnea had been progressive for the preceding six months and was now occurring at rest. A porcine aortic prosthesis had been implanted seven years before.

Physical examination revealed a harsh Grade IV/VI systolic ejection murmur at the left sternal border with radiation to the neck. Bibasilar rales were present.

ECHOCARDIOGRAPHY AND DOPPLER FINDINGS

M-mode and two-dimensional echocardiography revealed the porcine aortic prosthesis to be markedly thickened and probably calcified.

Left ventricular function was normal. A continuous-wave Doppler tracing from the right parasternal window is shown in Figure 60.

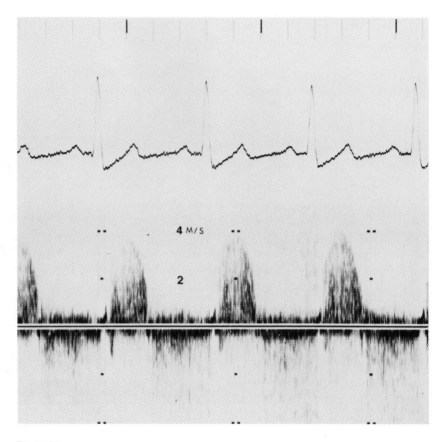

FIGURE 60.

What is the maximum velocity? _____

What is the gradient? _____

What is the diagnosis? _____

What is the treatment? _____

ANSWER

In the absence of a significant increase in left ventricular outflow tract velocities, the peak calculated transvalvular gradient is approximately 64 mm Hg. Note the late peak and prolonged ejection time characteristic of aortic stenosis.

At cardiac catheterization the prosthetic valve was unable to be crossed to measure a gradient. Successful replacement of a calcified, stenotic valve was undertaken the following morning.

Case #2

HISTORY AND PHYSICAL EXAMINATION

A 58-year-old female was admitted to the hospital with pulmonary edema. A Bjork-Shiley aortic prosthesis had been placed three years earlier and the patient had been essentially asymptomatic until one week prior to admission. Subsequent progressive shortness of breath prompted admission.

Physical examination revealed a tachypneic elderly woman. A Grade IV/VI systolic ejection murmur was heard at the base of the heart with radiation to the neck. A prosthetic closing sound was faintly heard.

ECHOCARDIOGRAPHY AND DOPPLER FINDINGS

M-mode and two-dimensional echocardiographic examinations were technically difficult. Continuous-wave Doppler of the aortic valve from the cardiac apex is shown in Figure 61.

Pulsed Doppler from the cardiac apex revealed aortic regurgitation evident less than 2 cm into the left ventricular chamber. Continuous-wave Doppler from the right parasternal region and suprasternal notch revealed velocities similar to those shown in Figure 61.

What is the peak aortic valve velocity? _____

What is the gradient? _____

What is the diagnosis? _____

ANSWER

The recording in Figure 61 shows peak velocities of 2.2 m/sec, indicating a transvalvular gradient of approximately 20 mm Hg, which is normal for this valve. Note the early onset of peak velocity. Valvular

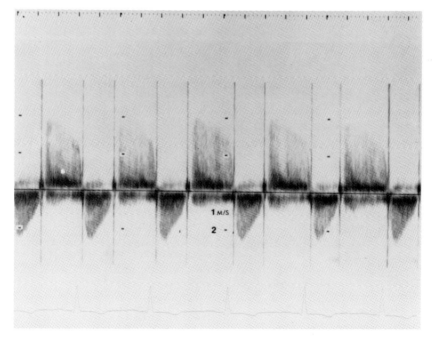

FIGURE 61.

regurgitation is minimal. Cardiac enzymes and subsequent catheterization revealed an acute anterior myocardial infarction secondary to occlusion of the anterior descending coronary artery. The prosthetic heart valve was normal.

Case #3

HISTORY AND PHYSICAL EXAMINATION

A 59-year-old female entered the emergency room because of transient blindness. She had had a Starr-Edwards mitral valve for ten years. She had no other symptoms.

On examination, her prosthetic clicks were loud and metallic. A soft diastolic rumble was present.

Two-dimensional (Figure 62A) and Doppler (Figure 62B) examinations were ordered to rule out prosthetic obstruction.

What is the maximal velocity? _____

What is the pressure halftime? _____

What is the orifice? _____

Is the valve obstructed? _____

ANSWER

This tracing demonstrates a normal prosthetic mitral valve. Maximal velocity is mildly elevated at 1.5 m/sec. Pressure halftime is 60 msec. When calculating the orifice area of prosthetic mitral valves, it is important to evaluate only the blood velocity profile. The earliest recorded diastolic velocity on this tracing represents the opening motion (opening click = OC) of the prosthetic disc. Including this artifact in the pressure halftime calculation would raise the maximal velocity to unacceptable limits and prolong the pressure halftime by 100 msec, creating a false picture of mitral stenosis. While it is important to exclude the valve motion artifact from calculations when evaluating mechanical prosthetic valves, artifacts are useful for timing valve motion and the cardiac cycle.

Case #4

HISTORY AND PHYSICAL EXAMINATION

A 47-year-old white female with a history of mitral valve replacement was admitted for prolonged fever and malaise after a tooth extraction. She was started on broad-spectrum antibiotics pending the results of blood cultures. The patient continued to be febrile and two days later developed a loud holosystolic murmur. M-mode echocardiography of the mitral valve is shown in Figure 63, continuous-wave Doppler of transmitral flow in Figure 64, and pulsed Doppler at the posterior left atrial wall in Figure 65.

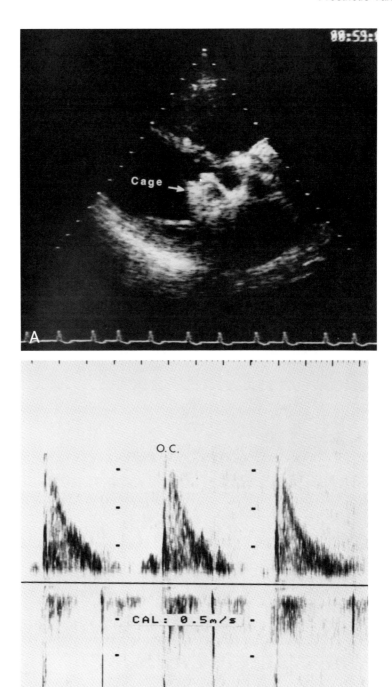

FIGURE 62.

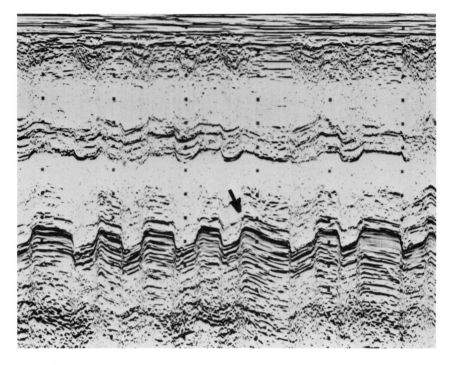

FIGURE 63.

Is there evidence of valve obstruction? _____

How severe is the regurgitation? _____

What is the most likely cause for these findings? _____

ANSWER

This patient has prosthetic valve endocarditis. The rounded early diastolic "hump" seen in the M-mode tracing is a nonspecific finding in prosthetic valve obstruction. Pressure halftime is diminished in Figure 64 and, more importantly, severe mitral regurgitation is indicated by pulsed-Doppler mapping of the regurgitant jet back to the posterior left atrial wall.

Case #5

HISTORY AND PHYSICAL EXAMINATION

A 65-year-old man was admitted to the hospital for evaluation of increasing dyspnea on exertion. He had had a Bjork-Shiley prosthesis placed in the mitral position four years before to correct mitral stenosis. He had done relatively well until two months prior to admission when he began noticing limitation in his ability to exercise, due to shortness

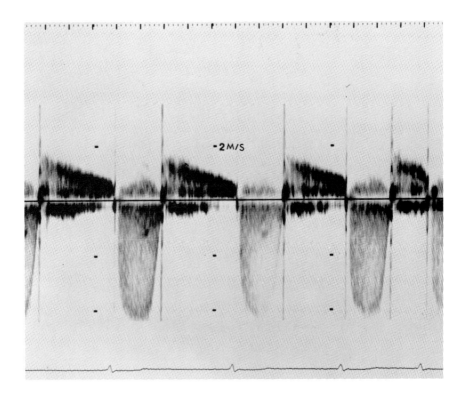

-2 M/S

FIGURE 64.

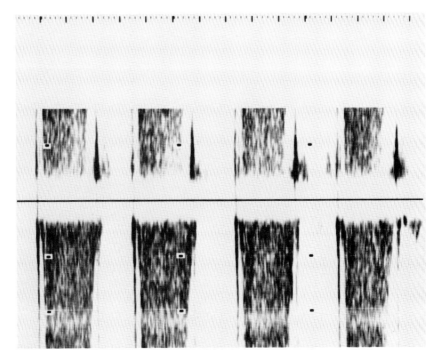

FIGURE 65.

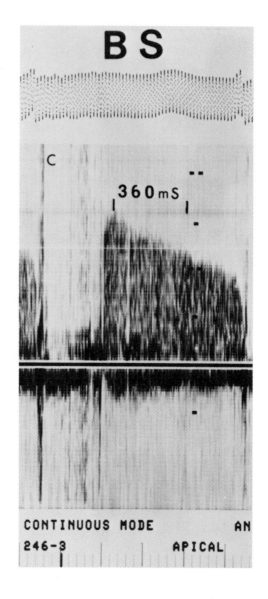

FIGURE 66.

of breath. This had progressed to shortness of breath after a walk of 100 feet or less.

Physical examination revealed a healthy appearing male in no acute distress. His heart rate was 84 and regular. His carotid pulses were brisk. His lungs were clear. His first heart sound revealed a loud prosthetic click. No systolic murmur was audible. The second heart sound was normal. No diastolic murmur was audible, and there were no gallops.

Two-dimensional echocardiography and fluoroscopy were normal. A continuous-wave tracing of the mitral valve diastolic flow is shown in Figure 66.

What is the diagnosis? _____

What is the calculated valve orifice area? _____

What is the next procedure to be done? _____

ANSWER

   This patient represents an example of subtle prosthetic valve dysfunction. Although the clinical examination, echocardiography, and fluoroscopy were normal, the Doppler study revealed severe mitral stenosis. The calculated valve orifice area is 0.65 cm^2.

   Although controversy exists as to the next procedure of choice, the patient was taken to surgery where a fibrosed thrombus was found almost totally occluding the atrial surface of his Bjork-Shiley valve. The valve was replaced, and the patient's symptoms disappeared. In this case, the patient did not undergo right and left heart catheterization or contrast injections prior to surgery. Experience has shown that invasive procedures may delay surgical correction of the valve and are associated with significant morbidity in patients with prosthetic dysfunction. The calculated orifice area of this valve was well below normal, and a decision was made to take the patient immediately to surgery. In cases where the diagnosis is less clear, documentation of the lesion by cardiac catheterization is indicated.

References

Caputo, G., Pearlman, A., Namay, D., and Dooley, T.: Detection of prosthetic valve incompetence using pulsed Doppler echocardiography. Circulation, *62*:III-252, 1980. (Abstract).

Ferrara, R.P., Labovitz, A.J., Wiens, R.D., Kennedy, H.L., and Williams, G.A.: Prosthetic mitral regurgitation detected by Doppler echocardiography. Am. J. Cardiol., *55*:229-230, 1985.

Hatle, L., and Angelsen, B.: Doppler Ultrasound in Cardiology: Physical Principles and Clinical Applications, 121-126. Philadelphia, Lea & Febiger, 1982.

Holen, J., Simonsen, S., and Froysaker, T.: An ultrasound Doppler technique for the non-invasive determination of the pressure gradient in the Bjork-Shiley mitral valve. Circulation, *59*:436-442, 1979.

Kotler, M., Mintz, G., Panidis, I., Morganroth, J., Segal, B., and Ross, J.: Non-invasive evaluation of normal and abnormal prosthetic valves. J. Am. Coll. Cardiol., *2*:151-173, 1983.

Mintz, G., Carlson, E., and Kotler, M.: Comparison of non-invasive techniques in evaluation of the non-tissue cardiac valve prosthesis. Am. J. Cardiol., *49*:39-44, 1982.

Nitter-Hauge, S.: Doppler echocardiography in the study of patients with mitral disc valve prostheses. Br. Heart J., *51*:61-69, 1984.

Panidis, I.P., Ross, J., and Mintz, G.S.: Normal and abnormal prosthetic valve function as assessed by Doppler echocardiography. J. Am. Coll. Cardiol., *8*:317-326, 1986.

Ryan, T., Armstrong, W.F., Dillon, J.C., and Feigenbaum, H.: Doppler echocardiographic evaluation of patients with porcine mitral valves. Am. Heart J., *111*:237-244, 1986.

Sagar, K.B., Wann, S., Paulsen, W.H.J., and Romhilt, D.W.: Doppler echocardiographic evaluation of Hancock and Bjork-Shiley prosthetic valves. J. Am. Coll. Cardiol., *7*:681–687, 1986.

Weinstein, I., Marberge, J., and Perez, J.: Ultrasonic assessment of the St. Jude prosthetic valve: M-mode, 2-dimensional, and Doppler echocardiography. Circulation, *68*:897–905, 1983.

Wilkins, G.T., Gillam, L.D., Kritzer, G.L., Levine, R.A., Palacios, I.F., and Weyman, A.E.: Validation of continuous-wave Doppler echocardiographic measurements of mitral and tricuspid prosthetic valve gradients: A simultaneous Doppler-catheter study. Circulation, *74*:786–795, 1986.

Williams, G.A., and Labovitz, A.L.: Doppler hemodynamic evaluation of prosthetic (Starr-Edwards and Bjork-Shiley) and bioprosthetic (Hancock and Carpentier-Edwards) cardiac valves. Am. J. Cardiol., *56*:325–332, 1985.

8

Left Ventricular Function

Cardiac Output

Recent studies have shown that the measurement of cardiac output (CO) by Doppler compares well to results obtained by invasive means (Figure 67). Sampling sites from which cardiac output measurements have been obtained include:

Ascending and descending aorta from the suprasternal notch
Apical mitral valve and tricuspid valve
Left ventricular outflow tract
Parasternal pulmonary artery

For any given window, the stroke volume (SV) is calculated as the product of the cross-sectional area of the valve or vessel through which the blood is flowing (CSA) and the flow velocity integral (FVI):

$$SV = CSA \times FVI$$

The cardiac output is then obtained by multiplying the stroke volume by the heart rate:

$$CO = SV \times HR$$

Flow Velocity Integral

The FVI is the product of the mean velocity and the time and is measured as the area under a specific cardiac complex of the Doppler spectral velocity display (Figure 68). It is directly proportional to the stroke volume and is expressed in units of distance (centimeters). For this reason, it is sometimes referred to as "stroke distance." The FVI

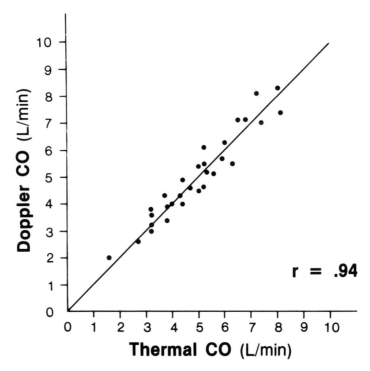

FIGURE 67. Comparison of thermodilution-determined cardiac output (CO) and Doppler-determined cardiac output as the average of multiple site determinations.

can be calculated using a commercially available digitizing computer or estimated by the following equation:

$$FVI = \frac{PV \times ET}{2}$$

where: PV = Peak velocity in cm/sec
ET = Ejection time in seconds

This equation usually underestimates the true FVI and should be recognized as only an estimate.

Cross-Sectional Area

The cross-sectional area is calculated for the site at which flow is measured. It is usually obtained by measuring the diameter (D) of the vessel or orifice involved and applying the equation:

$$CSA = \pi (D/2)^2 = 0.785 \ D^2$$

where π is approximately 3.14.

In determining the cardiac output from aortic flow, the diameter is usually measured at either the aortic valve anulus or the sinotubular junction, 3–5 cm above the aortic valve (Figure 69).

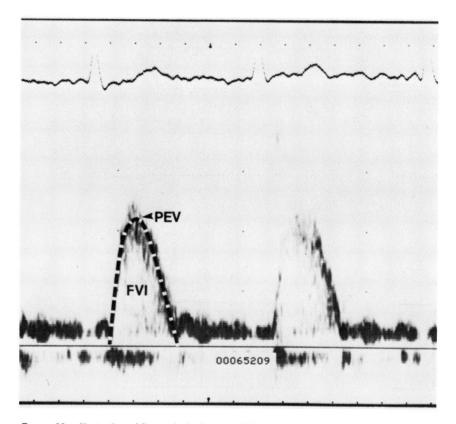

FIGURE 68.   Illustration of flow velocity integral (FVI) and peak ejection velocity (PEV) from ascending aortic velocity recording.

Examples

Figures 70–72 show examples of cardiac output calculations.

Relative Cardiac Output

The major source of error in the calculation of absolute cardiac output by Doppler is the measurement of the cross-sectional area. To compare changes over time in stroke volume or cardiac output in the same individual, however, the cross-sectional area need not be calculated since the change in the measured velocity integral is directly proportional to the change in stroke volume.

There are two major limitations in the use of Doppler-derived cardiac outputs. First, these calculations are not valid across a stenotic or insufficient valve because increases in velocity in the vicinity of an abnormal valve produce a false increase in the calculated integral. Second, the diameter used in the calculation of the cross-sectional area may be difficult to measure accurately. Any error is magnified because the diameter is squared in the area calculation.

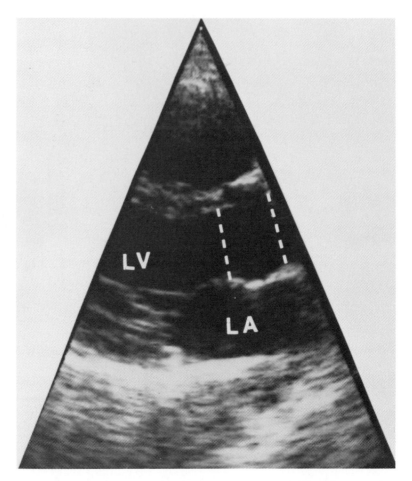

FIGURE 69. The two commonly used sites for measurement of aortic diameter and cross-sectional area for cardiac output determination.

Clinical Applications

Doppler measurements of the components of cardiac output have been shown to have several important clinical applications:

Evaluation of therapeutic intervention
Evaluation of pacemaker hemodynamics
Shunt calculations
Change in cardiac output with exercise
Regurgitation fractions

Evaluation of Therapeutic Intervention

The ability to follow an individual serially potentially eliminates the error of measuring cross-sectional area in determining a therapeutic effect on left ventricular performance. Several studies have demon-

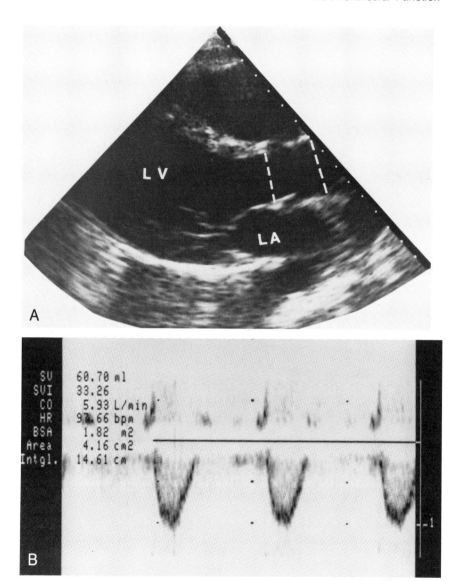

FIGURE 70. With an aortic anulus diameter of 2.3 cm (A), a flow velocity integral (Intgl) of 14.61 cm, and a heart rate of 97.6 bpm, the calculated cardiac output from the apical LVOT is 5.93 L/min (B).

strated significant changes in Doppler-measured flow velocity integrals following the administration of certain drugs, e.g., Dobutamine and nitroglycerine (Figure 73).

Evaluation of Pacemaker Hemodynamics

The ability of Doppler to provide a portable noninvasive method to objectively assess ventricular performance has been the basis of several investigations of optimal pacemaker hemodynamics. Doppler echocardiography has been shown to help predict which patients will benefit

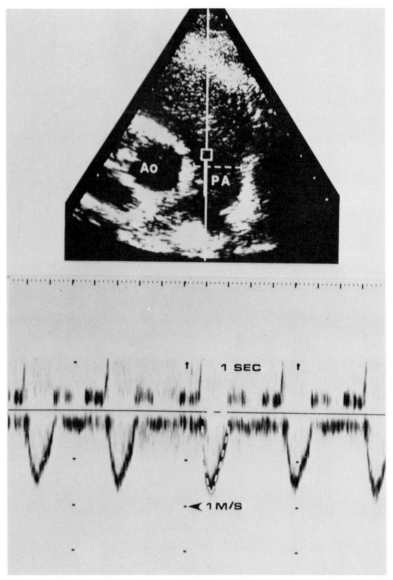

FIGURE 71.   Doppler determination of cardiac output from the main pulmonary artery (PA).
PA diameter = 2.0 cm
CSA = $0.785D^2$ = 3.14 cm^2
FVI = 11.7 cm
SV = FVI × CSA = 11.7 × 3.14 = 36.7 ml
Heart rate (HR) = 74 bpm
Cardiac output = HR × SV = 74 × 36.7 = 2.7 L/min

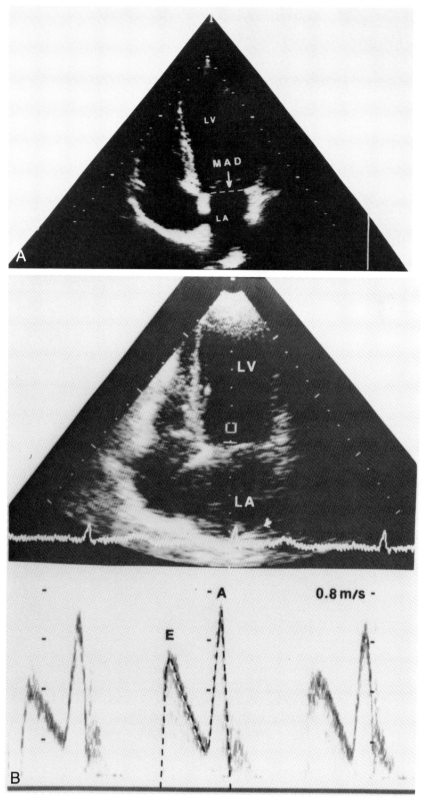

FIGURE 72. Doppler determination of cardiac output across the mitral valve. (A) Mitral anulus diameter (MAD) = 2.3 cm.
(B) FVI = 21.5 cm
HR = 70 bpm.
CO = FVI × CSA × HR = 21.5 × 4.16 × 70 = 6.3 L/min

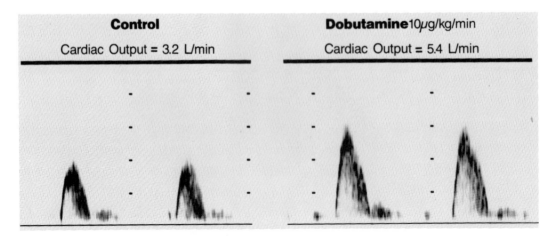

FIGURE 73. Recording from the suprasternal notch in a patient admitted to the cardiac care unit with an acute anterior myocardial infarction (left). After infusion of Dobutamine and an increase in the cardiac output from 3.2 to 5.4 L/Min, tracing (right) reflects a significant increase in stroke volume and cardiac output.

most from dual-chamber as opposed to ventricular-demand pacing modes. Recent studies suggest, in addition, that optimal atrioventricular delay may also be assessed by these means (Figures 74–76).

Doppler-Measured Regurgitant Fractions and Shunts

Doppler provides the ability to measure blood volume in many locations within the heart and great vessels. When normal flow is disrupted, as in intracardiac shunts and valvular regurgitant lesions, Doppler can theoretically identify and quantitate the disturbance by evaluation of volumes at serial points along the normal path of blood flow. Calculation of regurgitant volumes requires a measurement of volume across the regurgitant valve less the forward volume. For example, in a patient with mitral regurgitation:

$$\text{Regurgitant Fraction} = \frac{\text{Mitral SV} - \text{Aortic SV}}{\text{Mitral SV}}$$

In a similar way, the ratio of pulmonary to systemic flow (Q_p/Q_s) can be calculated by measuring right and left ventricular stroke volumes at the pulmonic and aortic valves, respectively. Mitral valve cardiac output can be substituted for pulmonary artery cardiac output in the presence of a ventricular septal defect to determine a left-to-right shunt.

Additional Parameters of Systolic Function

In addition to FVI measurement of stroke volume and cardiac output, a number of other Doppler parameters have been found useful in describing left ventricular systolic function. These include the peak ejection velocity (PEV), the pre-ejection period (PEP), left ventricular ejec-

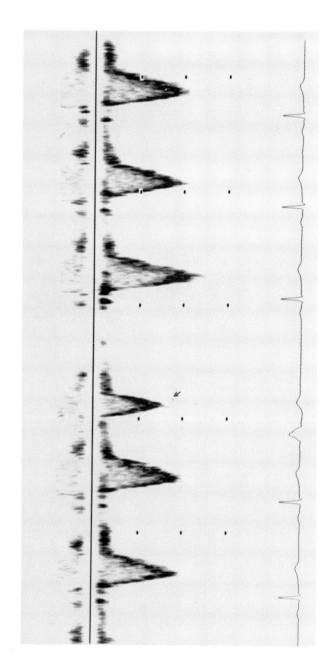

FIGURE 74. Beat-to-beat changes in stroke volume demonstrated with Doppler. Third beat from this LVOT recording is a PVC with an associated drop in stroke volume (arrow). However, the next, postextrasystolic, beat shows an augmentation in stroke volume.

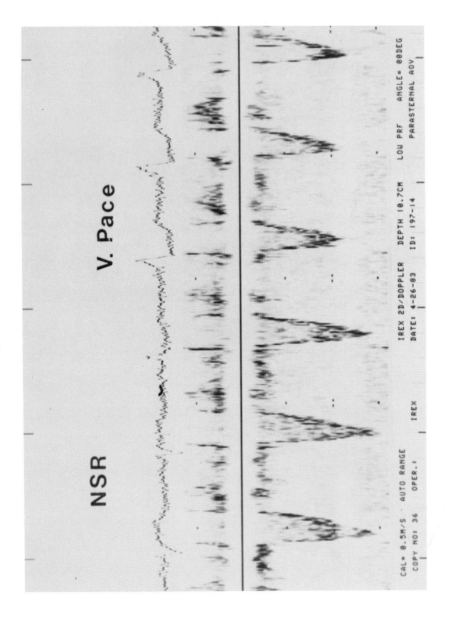

FIGURE 75. Tracing showing the sensitivity of Doppler in predicting which patients might be most sensitive to loss of AV synchrony. First three beats are normal sinus rhythm; last three beats are ventricular-paced beats. Note marked drop in stroke volume with ventricular pacing.

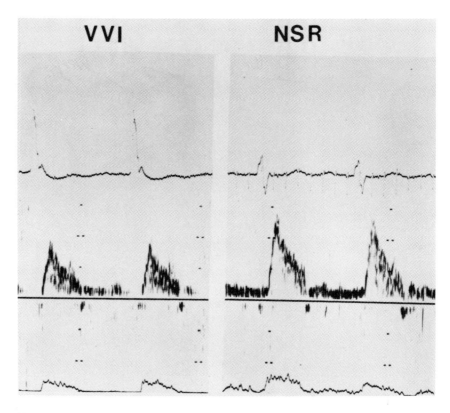

FIGURE 76.   Tracings for 73-year-old male with VVI pacer referred for evaluation of chronic congestive heart failure. At left, pulsed Doppler of the ascending aorta from suprasternal notch during ventricular demand pacing (VVI). At right, pacer inhibited (NSR); note 40% increase in stroke volume. Patient was treated by pacer reprogramming to a backup rate of 50 bpm, and congestive heart failure subsequently improved.

tion time (LVET), acceleration time (AT), and deceleration time (DT) (Figure 77).

Exercise Doppler

Initial experience with the measurement of Doppler FVIs from the suprasternal notch during both supine and upright exercise shows the potential value of this technique in evaluating left ventricular function with exercise. Figure 78A shows the response of a normal individual exhibiting a marked increase in cardiac output with exercise. Patients with left ventricular dysfunction or coronary artery disease frequently show a blunted response (Figure 78B).

Importantly, it appears feasible to measure these changes before and immediately after exercise, thus eliminating the potentially difficult task of acquiring information during exercise.

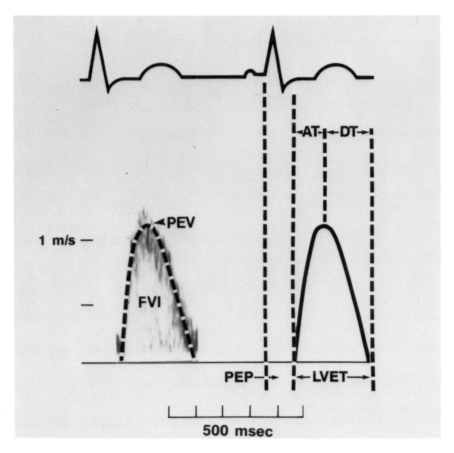

FIGURE 77. Parameters of left ventricular systolic function from aortic velocity tracing.

Diastolic Function

Recent studies have shown that detailed analysis of the velocity of left ventricular inflow as recorded by Doppler examination of transmitral flow may provide a clinically useful measure of left ventricular diastolic function (Figure 79). Doppler recordings of transmitral flow from the cardiac apex have a characteristic biphasic appearance. Two distinct peaks, representing early diastolic or passive filling velocities and late diastolic or atrial velocities, can be clearly identified. In normal individuals, the velocity of early diastolic filling (E) is equal to or greater than the velocity during atrial systole (A). In individuals with impaired diastolic function secondary to a variety of cardiovascular diseases, including hypertension, coronary artery disease, and left ventricular hypertrophy, there is a reversal of this ratio and a relative increase in the atrial component of diastolic filling velocities (Figure 80). Other parameters involving the use of the mitral filling contour, including the acceleration and deceleration halftimes, the ratio of the early diastolic integral to the atrial diastolic integral, and the 1/3 filling fraction, have been demonstrated to be impaired in individuals with acute and

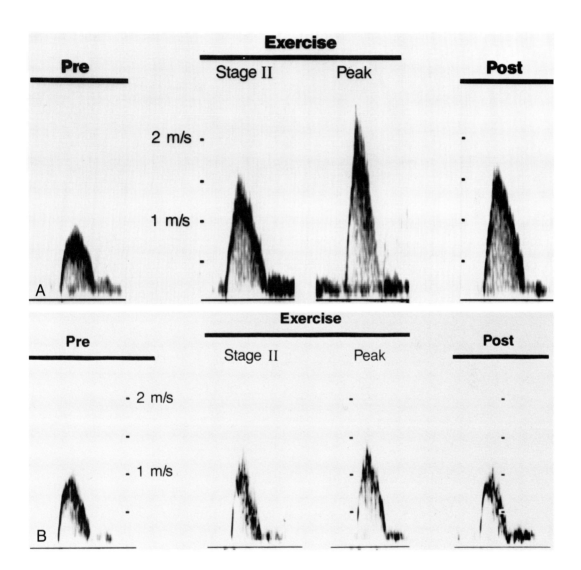

FIGURE 78.   Doppler spectral recordings of ascending aortic flow prior to (Pre), during (Stage II, Peak), and following (post) exercise in a normal individual (A) and in a patient with coronary artery disease (B). Note blunted velocity response in (B).

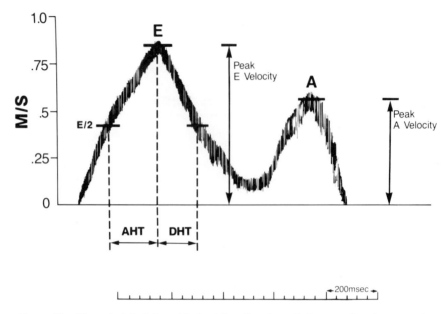

FIGURE 79. Characteristic left ventricular inflow Doppler velocity recording demonstrating early diastolic (E) and late diastolic (A) velocities, as well as acceleration (AHT) and deceleration (DHT) halftimes.

chronic coronary artery disease, hypertension, and ventricular hypertrophy (Figure 81).

References

Bryg, R.J., Labovitz, A.J., Mehdirad, A.A., Williams, G.A., and Chaitman, B.R.: Effect of coronary artery disease on Doppler-derived parameters of aortic flow during upright exercise. Am. J. Cardiol., *58*:14–19, 1986.

Chandrarathna, P.A.N., Nanna, M., McKay, C., Nimalasuriya, A., Swinney, R., Elkayam, U., and Rahimtoola, S.H.: Determination of cardiac output by transcutaneous continuous-wave ultrasonic Doppler computer. Am. J. Cardiol., *43*:234–237, 1984.

Elkayam, U., Gardin, J.M., Berkley, R., Hughes, C.A., and Henry, W.L.: The use of Doppler flow velocity measurements to assess the hemodynamic response to vasodilator in patients with heart failure. Circulation, *67*:377–383, 1983.

Fisher, D.C., Sahn, D.J., Friedman, M.J., Larson, D., Valdes-Cruz, L.M., Harowitz, S., Goldberg, S.J., and Allen, H.D.: The mitral valve orifice method for noninvasive 2-dimensional echo Doppler determinations of cardiac output. Circulation, *67*:872–877, 1983.

Friedman, B.J., Drinkovic, N., Miles, H., Shih, W-J., Mazzoleni, A., and DeMaria, A.N.: Assessment of left ventricular diastolic function: Comparison of Doppler echocardiography and gated blood pool scintigraphy. J. Am. Coll. Cardiol., *8*:1348–1354, 1986.

Gardin, J.M., Kozlowski, J., Dabestani, A., Murphy, M., Kusnick, C., Allfie, A., Russell, D., and Henry, W.L.: Studies of Doppler aortic flow velocity during supine bicycle exercise. Am. J. Cardiol., *57*:327–332, 1986.

Goldberg, S.J., Sahn, D.J., Allen, H.D., Valdes-Cruz, L.M., Hoenecke, H., and Carnahan, Y.: Evaluation of pulmonary and systemic blood-flow by 2-di-

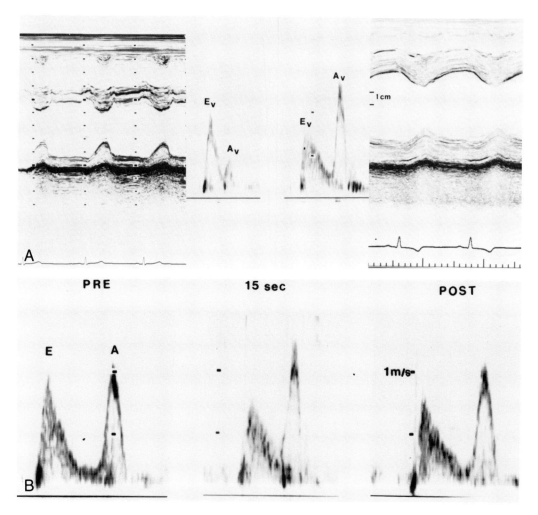

FIGURE 80. (A) In normal individuals (left), early diastolic velocity (E$_V$) is usually equal to or greater than late diastolic velocity (A$_V$). In individuals with less compliant ventricles, e.g., due to left ventricular hypertrophy (right), E/A ratio may be reversed. (B) Dramatic reversal of E/A ratio during myocardial ischemia, as demonstrated experimentally during coronary angioplasty, within 15 seconds of balloon inflation.

mensional Doppler echocardiography using fast Fourier transform spectral analysis. Am. J. Cardiol., *50:*1394–1400, 1982.

Huntsman, L.L., Gams, E., Johnson, C.C., and Fairbanks, M.S.: Transcutaneous determination of aortic blood-flow velocities in man. Am. Heart J., *89*:605–612, 1975.

Labovitz, A.J., Buckingham, T.A., Habermehl, K., Nelson, J., Kennedy, H.L., and Williams, G.A.: The effect of sampling site on the 2-dimensional echo Doppler determination of cardiac output. Am. Heart J., *109*:327–332, 1985.

Labovitz, A.J., Redd, R., Williams, G.A., and Kennedy, H.L.: The non-invasive assessment of pacemaker hemodynamics by Doppler echocardiography: Importance of left atrial size. J. Am. Coll. Cardiol., *6*:196–200, 1985.

Lewis, J.F., Kuo, L.C., Nelson, J.G., Limacher, M.C., and Quinones, M.A.: Pulsed Doppler echocardiographic determination of stroke volume and cardiac output: Clinical validation of two new methods using the apical window. Circulation, *70*:425–431, 1984.

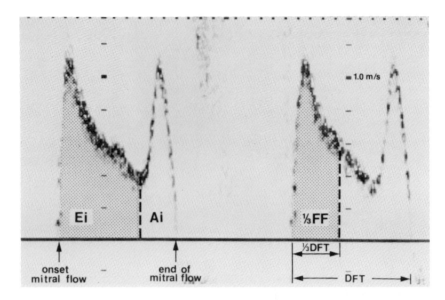

FIGURE 81. Additional derived parameters for evaluation of left ventricular diastolic filling include ratios of time velocity integrals in early (Ei) and late diastolic (Ai), and ratio of integral of the first third of diastole to total velocity integral (1/3 filling fraction).

Magnin, P.A., Stewart, J.A., Myers, S., VonRomm, O., and Kisslo, J.A.: Combined Doppler and phased array echocardiographic estimation of cardiac output. Circulation, *63*:388–392, 1981.

Mehdirad, A.A., Williams, G.A., Labovitz, A.J., Bryg, R.J., and Chaitman, B.R.: Evaluation of left ventricular function during upright exercise: Correlation of exercise Doppler with post-exercise two-dimensional echocardiography. Circulation, *75*:413–419, 1987.

Rokey, R., Kuo, L.C., Zoghbi, W.A., Limacher, M.C., and Quinones, M.A.: Determination of parameters of left ventricular diastolic filling with pulsed Doppler echocardiography: Comparison with cineangiography. Circulation, *71*:543–550, 1985.

Sabbah, H.N., Khaja, F., Brymer, J.F., McFarland, T.M., Albert, D.E., Snyder, J.E., Goldstein, S., and Stein, P.D.: Noninvasive evaluation of left ventricular performance based on peak aortic blood acceleration measured with a continuous-wave Doppler velocity meter. Circulation, *74*:323–329, 1986.

Sanders, P.S., Yeager, S., and Williams, R.G.: Measurement of systemic and pulmonary blood-flow and Q_P/Q_S ratio using Doppler and 2-dimensional echocardiography. Am. J. Cardiol., *51*:952–956, 1983.

Snider, A.R., Gidding, S.S., Rocchini, A.P., et al.: Doppler evaluation of left ventricular diastolic filling in children with systemic hypertension. Am. J. Cardiol., *56*:921–926, 1985.

Spirito, P., Maron, B.J., and Bonow, R.O.: Noninvasive assessment of left ventricular diastolic function: Comparative analysis of Doppler echocardiographic and radionuclide angiographic techniques. J. Am. Coll. Cardiol., *7*:518–526, 1986.

9

Congenital Heart Disease in the Adult

Ventricular Septal Defect

The finding of a high velocity jet within the right ventricle during systole is virtually diagnostic of ventricular septal defect. The jet should be found above the tricuspid valve during systole and be oriented in a direction away from the right atrium to avoid confusion with tricuspid regurgitation. Parasternal, apical, and subcostal windows are all useful in describing this lesion. The ability to simultaneously image the defect is helpful. However, because of the small size of many ventricular septal defects, the Doppler signal is frequently found in the absence of a visible defect. Increased velocity and turbulence of pulmonic flow are associated findings in the presence of a significant ventricular septal defect. Figure 82 is an example of a ventricular septal defect.

Atrial Septal Defect

The flow across an atrial septal defect is of considerably lower velocity than across a ventricular septal defect, usually ranging from 0.25 to 1.0 m/sec. The Doppler signal is characterized as flow across the atrial septum throughout the cardiac cycle. It is usually best recorded in the short-axis or subcostal views. Increased pulmonic flow is an associated finding in the presence of a significant shunt. Figure 83 is a characteristic recording of an atrial septal defect obtained from the parasternal short-axis window.

Coarctation of the Aorta

Coarctation of the aorta is an uncommon cause of hypertension in the adult. This lesion is characterized by Doppler as an increased ve-

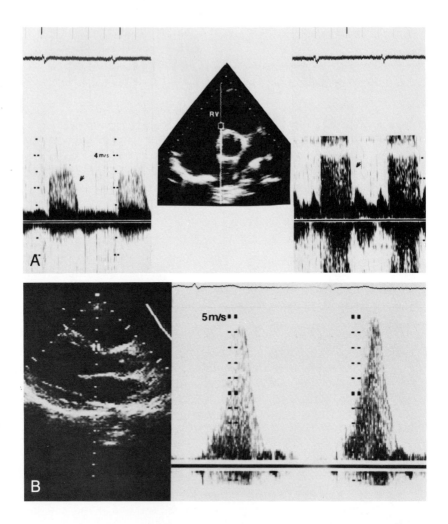

FIGURE 82. Ventricular septal defect in the short-axis view. (A) Continuous-wave Doppler (left) shows high velocity systolic flow toward the transducer. Pulsed Doppler (right) localizes the origin of the jet as aliased signals at the septal level. (B) The parasternal long-axis view is also useful as shown in this example of high velocity jet moving from left ventricle to right ventricle during systole.

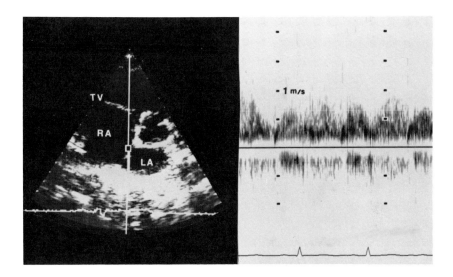

FIGURE 83. Atrial septal defect from parasternal short-axis window. Pulsed-mode sample volume is placed in the area of the atrial septum (left). Doppler signal (right) reveals continuous phasic velocities toward the transducer. This flow should be carefully documented by observing it on both sides of the atrial septum to distinguish it from normal vena cava flow.

locity in the descending aorta from the suprasternal window. The Bernoulli equation can be used to estimate the gradient across the coarctation. Figure 84A reveals a calculated 44-mm Hg gradient across the coarctation in a continuous-wave tracing. Figure 84B shows pulsed Doppler above and below the coarct site.

Patent Ductus Arteriosus

These relatively rare lesions in the adult can be recorded by Doppler either from the pulmonary artery or, less commonly, the aorta. In the pulmonary artery, the two characteristic findings are: 1) increased systolic velocities and, more importantly, 2) prominent diastolic flow, not seen in the right ventricular outflow tract. This diastolic flow must be distinguished from pulmonic regurgitation by the absence of diastolic flow on the ventricular side of the pulmonic valve (Figure 85).

Doppler can be used to confirm echocardiographic findings in this disease.

References

Daniels, O., Hopman, J.C.W., Stelinga, G.B.A., Busch, H.J., and Peer, P.G.M.:
Doppler flow characteristics in the main pulmonary artery and A/Ao ratio

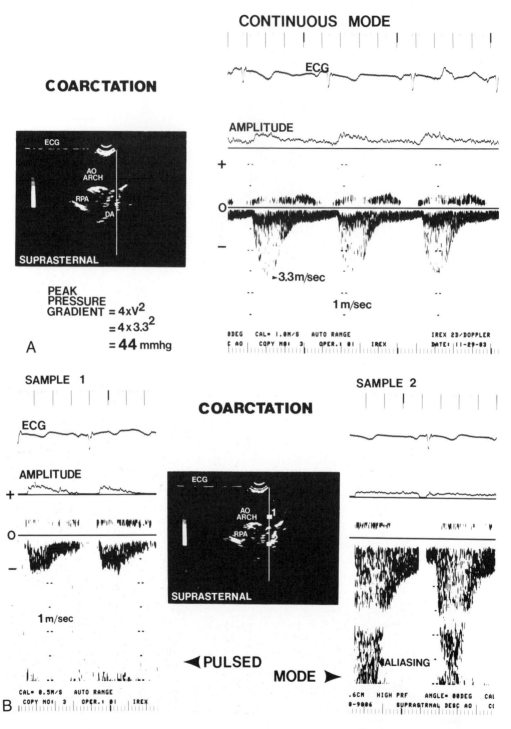

CONTINUOUS MODE

ECG

AMPLITUDE

COARCTATION

ECG
AO ARCH
RPA
DA
SUPRASTERNAL

+

O

−

►3.3m/sec

1 m/sec

PEAK
PRESSURE
GRADIENT $= 4 \times V^2$
$= 4 \times 3.3^2$

A $= 44$ mmhg

0DEG   CAL= 1.0M/S   AUTO RANGE   IREX 2D/DOPPLER
C AO   COPY NO: 3   OPER.: 01   IREX   DATE: 11-29-83

SAMPLE 1

ECG

AMPLITUDE
+

O

−

COARCTATION

ECG
AO ARCH
RPA
SUPRASTERNAL

SAMPLE 2

1 m/sec

CAL= 0.5M/S   AUTO RANGE
B   COPY NO: 3   OPER.: 01   IREX

◄ PULSED
MODE ►

ALIASING

.6CM   HIGH PRF   ANGLE= 00DEG   CAL
0-9006   SUPRASTERNAL DESC AO   C(

FIGURE 84.   A. Two-dimensional echo (left) and continuous-wave Doppler (right) of a coarctation of the aorta. Suprasternal notch echocardiogram shows brightness and apparent narrowing at the level of the pulmonary artery. Coarctation is confirmed by the high velocity jet away from the transducer through the same area. B. Pulsed-mode Doppler of coarctation. Typical aortic flow velocities appear above the coarctation (left). Aliasing below the coarct (right) is compatible with the high velocity flow jet.

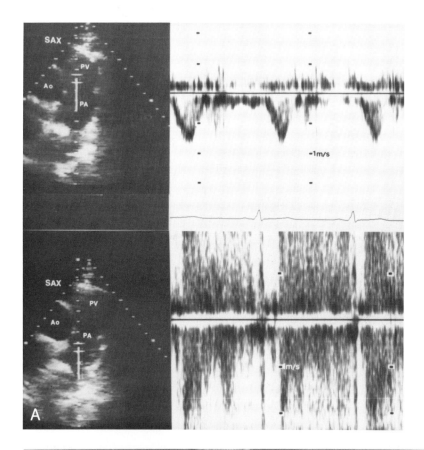

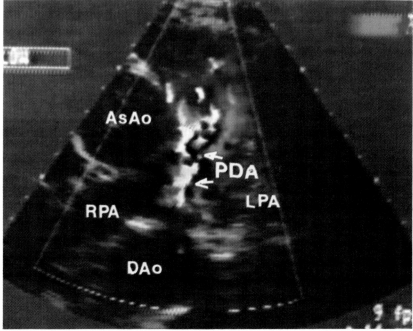

FIGURE 85.   Patent ductus arteriosus. (A) Doppler examination of the right ventricular outflow tract (top) shows only systolic velocities. Pulmonary artery tracing (bottom) shows both systolic velocities and a diastolic flow disturbance. (B) Color flow recording demonstrates the flow from descending aorta (DAo) to pulmonary artery through the patent ductus (PDA).

before and after ductal closure in healthy newborns. Pediatric Cardiol., *3*:99–104, 1982.

Hatle, L., and Rokseth, R.: Non-invasive diagnosis and assessment of ventricular septal defect by Doppler ultrasound. Acta Med. Scand., *645*:47–56, 1981.

Johnson, S.L., Rubenstein, S., Kawabori, I., Dooley, D.K., and Baker, D.W.: The detection of atrial septal defect by pulsed Doppler flowmeter. Circulation, *68*:53–54, 1976. (Abstract)

Magherini, A., Azzolina, G., Wiechmann, V., and Fantini, F.: Pulsed Doppler echocardiography for diagnosis of ventricular septal defects. Br. Heart J., *43*:143–147, 1980.

Stevenson, J.G.: Echo Doppler analysis of septal defects. *In* Cardiovascular Applications of Doppler Echocardiography. Edited by P. Peronneau and B. Diebold. Paris Inserm., *111*:515–540, 1983.

Stevenson, J.G., Kawabori, I., Dooley, T., and Guntheroth, W.G.: Diagnosis of ventricular septal defect by pulsed Doppler echocardiography: Sensitivity, specificity and limitations. Circulation, *58*:322–326, 1978.

Stevenson, J.G., Kawabori, I., and Guntheroth, W.G.: Non-invasive detection of pulmonary hypertension in patent ductus arteriosus by pulsed Doppler echocardiography. Circulation, *60*:355–359, 1979.

10

Color Doppler Echocardiography

Basic Features

As described in Chapter 1, color Doppler echocardiography uses multigate Doppler to produce a visible "map" of flow within the heart and great vessels. To do this, Doppler machines analyze multiple points along a line of information generated by a single burst of ultrasound. Over 250,000 points are analyzed each second by an "autocorrelator." The autocorrelator compares the frequency of the returning signal with that of the original signal and assigns a color value to the difference. The color is displayed at its appropriate location on the screen. Alternate sweeps of ultrasound produce color maps and imaging information, and the image and color map are then superimposed. The result has been called a "noninvasive angiogram," simultaneously displaying anatomy and flow.

Technique

The technique of applying color Doppler is similar to that of both imaging echo and conventional Doppler. The transducer is placed in the usual parasternal and apical windows as for standard imaging. The color flow is turned on, and the signals are automatically displayed superimposed on the image. The transducer is then angulated to "optimize" the color display. In parasternal views, the final window is a compromise between optimal imaging and optimal Doppler. Apical windows often produce excellent displays with little adjustment.

Color Display

With most commercially available equipment, two colors, red and blue, are used for unaliased flow display. However, no convention standardizes what they represent. Most machines display flow toward the transducer as red, and flow away from the transducer as blue (Figure 86), but some do the reverse. Aliased flow is displayed as a mixture of colors, often with green or turquoise introduced to display "variance." The higher the velocity or "turbulence," the greater the variance, and the greater the admixture of yellow or turquoise. This display outlines areas of high velocity, and make them stand out to the viewer.

Color Doppler has, like other ultrasound techniques, both advantages and disadvantages.

Advantages

EFFICIENCY

One of the major advantages of color Doppler is the speed with which normal and abnormal flow can be identified. The ability to visualize moving cells makes regurgitant lesions or shunts quickly recognizable and facilitates localization for sampling with conventional pulsed and continuous-wave Doppler.

ACCURACY

Although its usefulness is still controversial, the color display of high velocity jets and regurgitant lesions may make it easier to align the

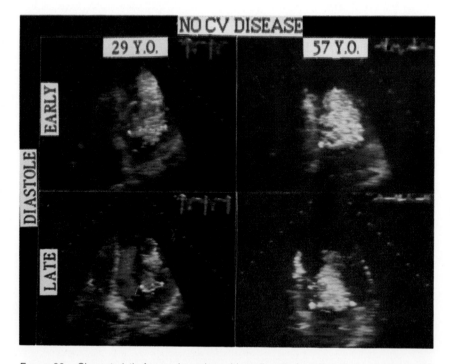

FIGURE 86. Characteristic frames in early and late diastole from the cardiac apex in a 29-year-old male (left) and a 57-year-old male (right). Early diastolic flow toward the transducer is displayed in red. Vertical flow away from the transducer toward the aortic valve, frequent in late diastole, is displayed in blue (lower left).

Doppler beam with the jet and may improve accuracy as well as efficiency.

GRAPHIC DISPLAY

One of the major difficulties of conventional Doppler and M-mode echocardiography is the need to understand what the tracings mean for appropriate interpretation, making it difficult to convey findings to others who may lack the necessary experience. Color Doppler is similar to other contrast techniques so that it makes data and spacial orientation easier to comprehend.

Disadvantages

Like all ultrasound, particularly conventional Doppler, color Doppler is limited to available windows and is sensitive to both depth of interrogation and misalignment of beam and flow. Also, the fact that flow mapping is a pulsed-Doppler technique imposes some disadvantages such as undesired aliasing.

ALIASING

Since the whole depth of the image may be sampled along 30 lines of information, the pulsed repetition frequency of the transducer must remain low, usually in the range of 4–8 kHz. A typical color Doppler display aliases at a blood velocity of 60 cm/sec. Aliasing can be both an advantage and a disadvantage. It can be useful in that it causes a reversal of color as it "wraps around" and outlines higher velocity flows. On the other hand, even normal velocities are above the sampling limits of the machine, and confusing patterns may result.

WALL MOTION

Doppler shifts are caused not only by flowing blood but by moving cardiac muscle and valves, which produce stronger returning signals than those from red cells. Various methods are used to reject these unwanted signals, based on echo signal strength, low velocity filters, or a combination of both.

SENSITIVITY AND GAIN DEPENDENCE

Because of the analysis technique and the volume of information processed, color Doppler has been less sensitive than conventional Doppler to weak signals. The display can be improved by turning up the color gain, but this introduces more noise into the display, which may mask a weak signal. Also, the returning signals may become displayed over a larger area, magnifying the apparent size of a signal source.

COMBINED LESIONS

Complex lesions may produce a multitude of flows in a small area in both systole and diastole. The result can be a confusion of color filling the screen, possibly hindering rather than helping an accurate diagnosis. Newer machines have reduced this problem by displaying flow only in one direction, or "moving the color baseline," effectively suppressing the flow display to one direction only.

QUANTITATION

All color Doppler machines display increasing flow velocity as gradients of color. However, color difference does not really correlate with difference in speed so that color values themselves can become difficult to differentiate. As a result, quantitation of velocity requires pulsed and continuous-wave Doppler.

FRAME RATE

The construction of a color flow image takes a great deal of time, dropping the frame rate as low as 10 frames per second.
This introduces the disadvantage of temporal ambiguity.

Applications

Stenotic Lesions

Color Doppler has theoretical advantages for the localization and quantitation of stenotic lesions. It visually displays the stenotic area and resultant jet as distinct from normal flow. However, it does have some practical limitations for this application. First, while it would be ideal to visualize and measure the stenotic orifice, the presence of calcification, the gain dependence of the display, and the problem of a simultaneous accurate imaging of the orifice (perpendicular beam orientation) and a Doppler signal (parallel orientation) often combine to prevent such measurements. When calcification is present, the color display often drops out of the image in the calcified area. The jet often diverges after leaving the orifice, precluding an accurate orifice measurement distal to the lesion. Turning up the gain to image within the calcified area often produces blooming of both the imaging and Doppler signals, obscuring the lesion. Also, as the transducer is angulated to improve the Doppler signal, the anatomic image becomes skewed and inaccurately displayed.

MITRAL STENOSIS

Color Doppler is particularly apt for acquiring information about mitral stenosis. Jet angulation can be identified, and the rapidity and accuracy of pulsed and continuous-wave Doppler sampling improved. The presence of associated mitral regurgitation is easily seen, and the jet of mitral stenosis can be quickly separated from coexisting aortic insufficiency.

AORTIC STENOSIS

Like imaging echocardiography, color Doppler easily confirms the presence of aortic stenosis, but quantitation of the orifice using flow mapping is also subject to the same limitations as imaging echocardiography, as well as others described above. In addition, the jet of aortic stenosis is rarely identified for beam orientation. Except in the suprasternal window, the jet is often not in the imaging plane. Aortic stenosis is therefore usually quantitated as described in Chapter 4.

TRICUSPID STENOSIS

Color Doppler can be extremely useful for diagnosing tricuspid stenosis. Documentation is often difficult from anatomic imaging or M-mode Doppler, but the presence of a narrowed, higher than normal velocity jet is easily recognized.

Insufficient Lesions

MITRAL INSUFFICIENCY

Mitral insufficiency is easily recognized when displayed on the screen (Figure 87). The presence of an aliased jet of blood in the normally colorless atrium during systole is diagnostic of this lesion. The jet may be seen from the parasternal long or short axis or from the apical windows. It is not uncommon to see it from only one or two windows. Quantitation has been attempted by evaluating the depth of the regurgitant flow or the area of the jet on the screen. Both techniques have been useful for qualitative evaluation but are limited by gain dependence and system sensitivity. A moderate lesion may not be seen or may appear insignificant if color gain is too low, and may appear to be severe if gain is turned up too high. General agreement exists that the gain should be just high enough to produce a small amount of background noise, and no more.

AORTIC INSUFFICIENCY

Aortic insufficiency is closer to the chest wall and easier to recognize than mitral insufficiency. A high velocity jet of blood above the mitral valve in diastole can be seen in all views: parasternal, short axis, and apical (Figure 88). Both the depth of penetration of the jet into the left ventricle and the size of the jet in the left ventricular outflow tract have been used to qualitatively assess the lesion.

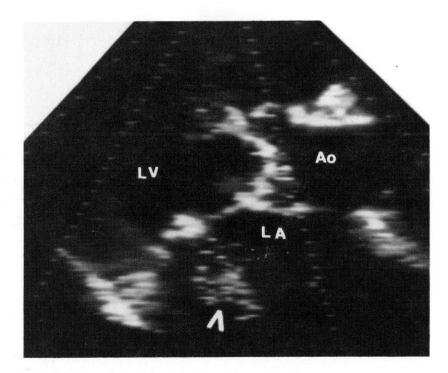

FIGURE 87. High velocity regurgitant jet of mitral insufficiency (arrow) is clearly seen in the left atrium.

TRICUSPID AND PULMONIC INSUFFICIENCY

Right-sided insufficient jets are a common finding in both color and conventional Doppler recordings in normal individuals. In color, only a small wisp is usually seen (Figure 89). More severe tricuspid insufficiency can fill the right atrium, as well as the inferior vena cava and hepatic veins, causing obvious systolic color flow (Figure 90).

Shunts

One of the potentially most valuable uses of color flow Doppler is the identification of intracardiac shunts.

VENTRICULAR SEPTAL DEFECTS

Ventricular septal defects, typically with high velocity flow, are readily identified by color techniques. The site and number of lesions can quickly be found, providing immediate clinically useful information (Figure 91).

ATRIAL SEPTAL DEFECT

Since lower velocities are present in the atria, atrial septal defects are more difficult to evaluate. The difficulty lies in distinguishing

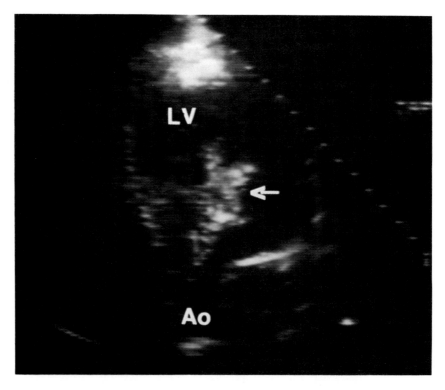

FIGURE 88. Apical five-chamber view illustrating high velocity diastolic jet (arrow) in an individual with moderate aortic insufficiency.

between the abnormal flow of an ASD and the normal flow from the inferior vena cava, which courses along the interatrial septum essentially in the same direction. To avoid false positive results, diagnosis should be reserved for the lesions in which bidirectional flow can be seen.

Prosthetic Valves

Color Doppler appears to be useful in the evaluation of prosthetic heart valves. While conventional pulsed and continuous-wave Doppler have rapidly become an integral part of the evaluation of patients with prosthetic valves, the eccentricity of both anterograde and insufficient jets limits the application of these techniques. Color Doppler allows rapid identification of the spacial orientation of blood flow through both disc and tissue prosthetic heart valves. Recent reports have suggested that color Doppler may be particularly helpful as a diagnostic aid in patients with paravalvular leak.

Summary

Color Doppler adds an understandable new dimension to the Doppler examination. It has the same limitations as conventional Doppler but

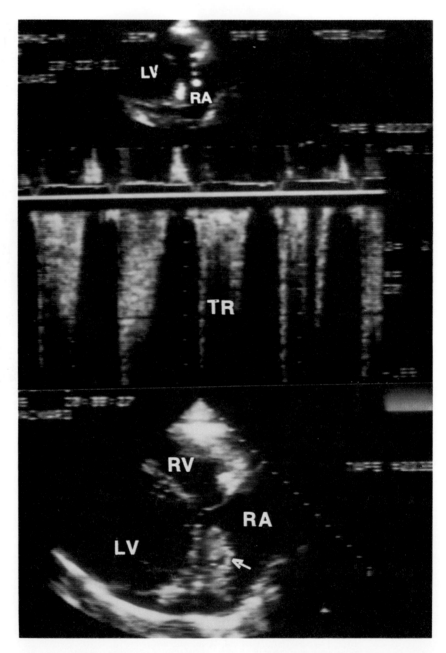

FIGURE 89.   With sampling in the right atrium (top), the typical systolic jet of tricuspid insufficiency is seen in both conventional Doppler (middle) and color flow imaging (bottom, arrow).

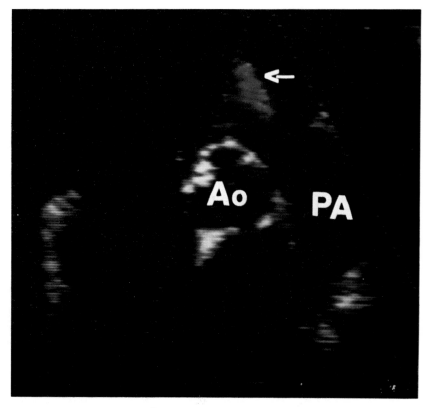

FIGURE 90. Lesion of pulmonic insufficiency demonstrated in color Doppler in a reddish view (arrow) of flow moving back across the pulmonic valve during diastole.

the advantage of a graphic display. It provides anatomically diagnostic and useful information quickly but cannot at present be used for exact quantitation of lesions.

References

Ludomirsky, A., Huhta, J.C., Vick, G.W., Murphy, D.J., Danford, D.A., and Morrow, W.R.: Color Doppler detection of multiple ventricular septal defects. Circulation, *74*:1317–1322, 1986.

Miyatake, K., Izumi, S., Okamoto, M., Kinoshita, N., Asonuma, H., Nakagawa, H., Yamamoto, K., Takamiya, M., Sakakibara, H., and Nimura, Y.: Semiquantitative grading of severity of mitral regurgitation by real-time two-dimensional Doppler imaging technique. J. Am. Coll. Cardiol., *7*:82–88, 1986.

Miyatake, K., Izumi, S., Shimizu, A., Kinoshita, N., Okamoto, M., Sakakibara, H., and Nimura, Y.: Right atrial flow topography in healthy subjects studied with real-time two-dimensional Doppler flow imaging technique. J. Am. Coll. Cardiol., *7*:425–431, 1986.

Omoto, R., Takamoto, S., Ueda, K., Namekawa, K., and Kondo, Y.: The development of real-time two-dimensional Doppler echocardiography and its clin-

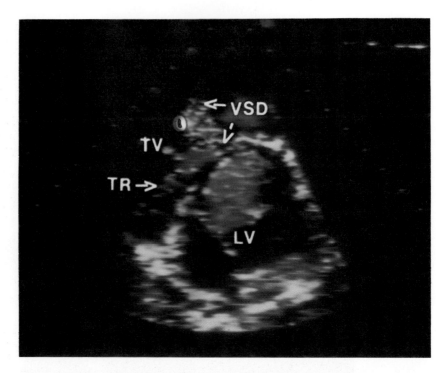

FIGURE 91.   Color Doppler during systole of patient with both a ventricular septal defect and tricuspid regurgitation. The two lesions are clearly separated.

ical significance in acquired valvular diseases with special reference to the evaluation of valvular regurgitation. Japanese Heart J., *25*:325–340, 1984.

Oritz, E., Robinson, P.J., Deanfield, J.E., Franklin, R., Macartney, F.J., and Wyse, R.K.H.: Localisation of ventricular septal defects by simultaneous display of superimposed colour Doppler and cross sectional echocardiographic images. Br. Heart J., *54*:53–60, 1985.

Suzuki, Y., Kambara, H., Kadota, K., Tamaki, S., Yamazato, A., Nohara, R., Osakada, G., and Kawai, C.: Detection and evaluation of tricuspid regurgitation using a real-time, two-dimensional, color-coded, Doppler flow imaging system: Comparison with contrast two-dimensional echocardiography and right ventriculography. Am. J. Cardiol., *57*:811–815, 1986.

Suzuki, Y., Kambara, H., Kadota, K., Tamaki, S., Yamazato, A., Nohara, R., Osakada, G., and Kawai, C.: Detection of intracardiac shunt flow in atrial septal defect using a real-time two-dimensional color-coded Doppler flow imaging system and comparison with contrast two-dimensional echocardiography. Am. J. Cardiol., *56*:347–350, 1985.

Glossary

Aliasing. Inappropriate (ambiguous) representation of velocities that exceed the measuring capacity of a pulsed-Doppler system. The velocity limit at which this occurs is defined by the pulse repetition frequency (PRF), the interrogating frequency (FO), and the range.

Angle of Incidence. Angle between the interrogating sound beam and the velocity vector of the blood flow. An angle of incidence greater than 20° significantly lowers the measured velocity and underestimates actual flow velocities.

Bandwidth. Difference between highest and lowest frequencies present. If frequencies from 200 to 500 Hz are present, the bandwidth is 300 Hz. On the spectral tracing, a widened bandwidth implies multiple velocities in the same sample volume or along the continuous wave beam path.

Bernoulli Equation. Hydraulic formula relating changes in pressure (gradient) across an obstruction to velocity change. $P_1 - P_2 = 4V^2$, see Chapter 3, "Calculations."

Chirp Z. Method of analyzing individual frequencies within a complex waveform. Chirp Z and FFT are the two commonly used analysis methods in Doppler echocardiography.

Continuous-Wave Doppler. Use of two transducers or sets of transducers to simultaneously send and receive ultrasound waves. Continuous-wave Doppler has no theoretical velocity limitations.

Disturbed (nonlaminar) Flow. Flow characterized by multiple directions and speeds of red blood cells, usually occurring in the presence of an obstruction to flow.

Doppler Effect. A change of frequency (and corresponding wavelength) from the original due to relative motion between source and reflector. Doppler echocardiography uses the change in frequency between the emitted and reflected sound to display and measure the velocity of blood within the heart and great vessels.

Doppler Shift (F$_D$). The difference between the interrogating frequency (F$_O$) and the received frequency. The shift frequency is proportional to the speed of the reflectors.

Duplex Scanning. Combined imaging and Doppler echocardiography with either simultaneous Doppler and image, or updated 2-dimensional still frames, to help guide the Doppler examination.

Fast Fourier Transformation (FFT). Method of determining and displaying component frequencies in a complex waveform, often used in spectral analysis.

Hertz (Hz). Unit of frequency (1 Hz = 1 cycle/sec). In ultrasound, expressed as kilohertz (kHz) for thousands of cycles per second, or megahertz (MHz) for millions of cycles per second.

High PRF. Use of increased pulsed repetition frequency (PRF) to measure velocities outside the limits of pulsed Doppler. PRF is increased two to four times, with proportionate increases in measurable velocity. Since multiple samples are within the heart, however, range ambiguity is introduced.

Interrogating Frequency (F$_O$). Sound frequency emitted by the transducer, base for computation of Doppler shift. Increasing F$_O$ reduces the velocity limit of pulsed Doppler at any depth.

Jet. Discrete area of very high velocities distal to an obstruction. The velocity is proportional to the pressure difference (gradient) across the obstruction.

Laminar Flow. Characteristic blood flow in smooth structures, defined by parallel direction and speed of flow of most red blood cells and producing a narrow spectral bandwidth.

Multigate Doppler. Analysis of more than one sample volume along the path of a single pulse of ultrasound, used in flow mapping.

Nyquist Limitation. Inability of pulsed Doppler to measure (resolve) frequencies of more than one half the PRF. The Nyquist frequency is defined as PRF/2.

Range. Distance from the transducer in cm.

Sample Volume. Region from which sound is analyzed in pulsed Doppler, defined by sample length (range gate) and the width and depth of the interrogating beam.

Spectral Analysis. Breaking a complex waveform into its component frequencies by either FFT or Chirp Z methods.

Spectral Tracing (graph). Display of all velocities present as a graph versus time.

Velocity. Describes speed and direction of motion. Doppler echocardiography measures velocity as speed toward or away from the transducer.

Velocity Limit. Fastest velocity measurable by pulsed Doppler. The velocity limit is defined by the PRF, F$_O$, and range.

Wall Filter. Eliminates low frequency Doppler shifts from the spectrum, improving the ability to ignore heart wall motion.

"Wrap Around." Characteristic of aliasing with unresolved velocities, producing the appearance of a cutoff profile with the velocities superimposed on the opposite side of the tracing.

Index

Page numbers in italics refer to figures.